What if . . .

Survival Guide

for Physicians

Ronald B. Goodspeed, MD, MPH, FACP, FACPE
President and CEO
Southcoast Hospitals Group
Fall River, New Bedford, and Wareham, Massachusetts

Bruce Y. Lee, MD, MBA
Assistant Professor of Medicine
Section of Decision Sciences
and Clinical Systems Modeling
University of Pittsburgh
Pittsburgh, Pennsylvania

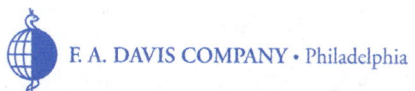
F. A. DAVIS COMPANY · Philadelphia

F. A. Davis Company
1915 Arch Street
Philadelphia, PA 19103
www.fadavis.com

Copyright © 2007 by F. A. Davis Company

Printed in the United States of America

Last digit indicates print number: 10 9 8 7 6 5 4 3 2 1

Acquisitions Editor: Andy McPhee
Manager of Content Development: Deborah Thorp
Developmental Editor: Brenna Mayer
Art and Design Manager: Carolyn O'Brien

As new scientific information becomes available through basic and clinical research, recommended treatments and drug therapies undergo changes. The author(s) and publisher have done everything possible to make this book accurate, up to date, and in accord with accepted standards at the time of publication. The author(s), editors, and publisher are not responsible for errors or omissions or for consequences from application of the book, and make no warranty, expressed or implied, in regard to the contents of the book. Any practice described in this book should be applied by the reader in accordance with professional standards of care used in regard to the unique circumstances that may apply in each situation. The reader is advised always to check product information (package inserts) for changes and new information regarding dose and contraindications before administering any drug. Caution is especially urged when using new or infrequently ordered drugs.

Library of Congress Cataloging-in-Publication Data
Goodspeed, Ronald B.
    What if . . . ? : survival guide for physicians / Ronald B.
Goodspeed, Bruce Y. Lee.
        p. ; cm.
    ISBN-13: 978-0-8036-1339-3
    ISBN-10: 0-8036-1339-3
    1.   Physicians—Life skills guides. 2.   Medical students—Life skills guides. 3.   Clinical competence. 4.   Medical emergencies. 5.   Physician and patient. I. Lee, Bruce Y. II. Title. III. Title: Survival guide for physicians.
    [DNLM: 1.   Clinical Competence. 2.   Emergencies. 3.   Emergency Treatment.
4.   Physician-patient Relations.   W 21 G655w 2007]
    R727 . G66 2007
    610—dc22
                                                                                                2006100697

This book is dedicated to

My wonderful wife, Karen; my editors, Andy McPhee and Brenna Mayer; and my co-author, Bruce. Their patience and invaluable help made it possible to complete this book. **R.G.**

My family, including my younger brother Tom, who left us far too soon; my close friends, who have stood by me through thick and thin; our editors, Andy and Brenna; and my co-author Ron—all of whom made it possible to complete this book. **B.L.**

Preface

Despite rigorous medical education and training, are medical students, residents, and physicians equipped to handle all the situations they may face? Over the course of our careers as practicing physicians, administrators, and educators, we've encountered a remarkable number of scenarios not covered by formal medical education and training. Some are common and others are unusual. Some are life-threatening and others aren't. However, all are important and potentially challenging. Whenever these scenarios occur, people usually assume that you can and will handle them—just because you are or will be a physician!

Through our book *What If...? Survival Guide for Physicians* we hope to fill some of these gaps in education and training and help physicians and students of all levels feel better prepared to handle whatever comes their way. Each entry in our book is similarly structured and presented, with sections on what to do in a given scenario and possible measures you can take to prepare for it or prevent it from happening. This structure makes it easy to absorb the straightforward, step-by-step instructions and tips on dealing with a variety of crises, such as:

- *What if a patient has a cockroach or similar insect in her ear canal?*
- *What if you have to deliver a baby outside the hospital?*
- *What if a patient threatens your life?*

There are also entries on less dangerous and more common situations for students, residents, and practitioners, such as:

- *What if you feel faint at the bedside or in the operating room?*
- *What if you have been up too many hours and are having trouble thinking?*
- *What if you think a patient is faking?*

Physicians at all levels, especially residents and medical students, typically have a driving need to feel knowledgeable and in control—even when their insides are swirling. This book can provide valuable tidbits of information that others around you may not know. Having such knowledge is empowering and fulfilling, and will help you become a confident, respected, and important source of information and experience to others. So, dive in and take your knowledge to another level!

Ronald B. Goodspeed
Bruce Y. Lee

Contents

First-Time Student Experiences

At the Bedside

What if ...

On the Hot Seat

What if ...

Student Life

What if ...

Emergency!

Health Care

What if ...

In the Field

What if ...

One-on-One Encounters

Patient

What if ...

Family or Friends
What if ...

Faraway Adventures
Wilderness
What if ...

What if . . . ?

First-Time
Student
Experiences

What if . . .

A patient or patient's family thinks you're a real doctor?

So, someone thinks you're a real doctor. After years of premedical and preclinical study, you probably think it feels good when someone calls you a doctor, listens to your clinical opinion, and depends on you. Think again.

Being a doctor carries a lot of responsibility. Will you be available on weekends or after hours? Are you prepared to take the blame if anything goes wrong, even if you weren't the cause? Can you answer all of the patient's questions? Can you take care of a life-threatening emergency? Are you prepared to deal with a patient who's angry, upset, delirious, or even violent? If the patient needs something, can you deliver it? Will you even be able to recognize when you're doing something wrong?

There are huge risks involved in pretending to be a doctor. You can injure or even kill a patient. You can hurt yourself physically and professionally. Without experience, you won't know what precautions to take or how to recognize dangerous situations. Even if no significant problems occur, if someone discovers your masquerade—and someone *will* discover it—you could fail your course and suffer significant disciplinary action. How will you be discovered? A patient might ask her nurse, physical therapist, or physician for you. When she's discharged from the hospital, she may ask for your office number or try to contact you later. There is a good chance that your advice to the patient will disagree with that of others. Even full-fledged physicians commonly disagree in their opinions. When these conflicts emerge, your team will soon realize the source of the conflicting advice.

Obviously, being a physician has its rewards. Why else would so many people go through all that training? However, until you're qualified and ready to handle the responsibilities and aggravations of a physician, you can't truly reap the rewards without problems quickly overpowering everything. So it's best not to pretend to be a doctor. You'll have plenty of time to be a real doctor in the future, and there are days when physicians long to be relatively responsibility-free medical students. So why rush it? Enjoy being a medical student while you can.

In fact, being a medical student has other advantages. You have time to focus on a few patients, listen to their concerns, provide emotional support, and identify clues and problems that the busy residents and attendings may miss. You don't need to be a full-fledged doctor to have an impact and earn the respect of patients.

What To Do

If someone mistakes you for a doctor, remind her that you're a medical student but feel free to explain what you can do for her. Take advantage of your status as a medical student. Show how important you can be. Be the patient's advocate. Promptly alert nurses and your team when the patient has a new medical problem. Spend time listening to your patient and her family. You can be an essential information source for your patient and your team.

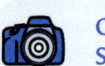 **CLINICAL SNAPSHOT**

Dangerous deception

As a medical student, you've been seeing a patient and his family every day for almost a week. Through hard work and attentiveness, you've built a rapport with them. One problem, though—they think you're his doctor. So, what happens if one day the patient starts having some chest pain? Can you tell if he's having a heart attack, angina, heart burn, pericarditis, an aortic dissection, or a panic attack? Do you know how to handle each of these problems?

The patient and his family will expect their "real doctor" to know what is going on and what to do. They'll be worried and may shower you with questions while you're trying to determine what to do. Do you try to handle the situation and risk seriously injuring or even killing the patient? Or do you get a "real doctor" to help and risk exposing your deception to the patient and his family and losing their trust? Don't get into this lose-lose situation. Don't pretend to be a doctor.

(Of course, make sure you know what you're talking about and don't mislead anyone.) Ask your residents and attending physicians how you can help your patient. Ask your patient and her family how you can help them. You'll be surprised at how much you can do. If you're honest, helpful, and attentive, patients and their families will depend on and respect you—everything that playing a doctor may have brought, but without all the dangers and hassles.

Prevention and Preparation

To avoid confusion about your role in a patient's health care, clearly introduce yourself as a medical student to the patient and her family. (Many times the attending or residents will do this for you.) Explain that, while you aren't yet a "real doctor," you're part of the team that is taking care of the patient and can serve as a liaison between the patient and the team. Be there when the patient needs something explained, has a concern, or needs comforting. You and the patient will soon learn how valuable a medical student can be.

What if . . .

You feel faint at the bedside or in the operating room?

Fainting, or *syncope,* is a common occurrence for first-time observers of procedures in the operating room (OR) or at the bedside. Feeling faint is the sensation of an impending loss of consciousness, characterized by feeling weak. Vision may be blurred, dim, or speckled with black spots. You may also experience *tinnitus.* If these symptoms are allowed to progress, a syncopal episode will ensue.

Syncope in a young healthy person is generally due to a transient decrease in blood pressure and subsequently diminished cerebral blood flow when sitting or standing. In a novice who's extremely worried about fainting or is experiencing severe emotional stress, vagus nerve activity can increase. This increased vagal activity can lead to bradycardia, accompanied by venous pooling in the lower extremities and hypotension, which commonly results in syncope. Fainting can be highly embarrassing and unpleasant. It also carries the potential for injury from falling—or injury to patients from falling on them!

What To Do

As soon as you start to feel faint, begin flexing and relaxing your leg muscles to enhance venous return to the heart. If you can, step away from the patient. Then try to squat down as promptly and tactfully as you can. The squat maneuver increases the venous return of blood to the heart, causing an override of the vagal activity and increasing your blood pressure and cerebral blood flow.

Depending on the circumstances, it may be more tactful to drop something on the floor, such as a pencil or an instrument, and then squat to pick it up. You might also squat to retie your shoelaces or straighten out your stockings or pant cuffs. Stay squatted as long as you can. Upon assuming the upright position, begin flexing and relaxing your leg muscles again. On rare occasions, the squat maneuver is inadequate but it may provide enough relief to excuse yourself from the room.

If you're gloved and "sterile," picking up things from the floor or tying your shoes isn't the best option. In that case, while flexing and relaxing your leg muscles, focus on the procedure you're observing. Imagine you're actually doing the procedure and try to anticipate the surgeon's next move.

 WARNING!!! Don't delay! At the first symptom, start your maneuvers to stop the vasovagal syncope cycle! Your safety and that of the patient is of the utmost importance. So, if your condition doesn't rapidly improve, set embarrassment aside and leave the room. Then lie down for a few minutes until you feel better. Although the recumbent position is the most effective treatment, it isn't as easily accomplished without excusing yourself from the procedure in progress.

Prevention and Preparation

Knowing what to do if you feel faint may be all you need to prevent it. Knowing that you can handle this situation if it develops is nearly always sufficient to prevent you from experiencing it. In addition, always make sure you're well hydrated and try not to begin the procedure on an empty stomach. Remember, now that you've read this *What if* scenario, you probably won't ever have this problem!

What if . . .

The first patient you're assigned to examine refuses?

You're about to examine your first real patient; your white coat is on, stethoscope somewhere on your body, and the history and physical script in your memory. Then, your first true foray into clinical medicine is derailed . . .

There are many reasons a patient may not allow you to examine her. The patient may not want to be seen by anyone other than the regular physician. Perhaps the patient wants to follow up on a previous conversation or discuss sensitive, confidential information. Commonly, patients don't want to spend time speaking to someone new, as they're late for a subsequent appointment, not in the appropriate mood, or suffering discomfort. Some patients associate being seen by a "trainee" or "student" with being used as a "teaching tool" or an "experimental subject."

Many patients also have their preferences and prejudices; so, unfortunately, some may be biased against you. In the eyes of the patient, you may not have the right appearance, race, or gender or be of the "right" age or physique. There are some situations in which such biases may be more prevalent. For example, male medical students may have more difficulty with female urology patients or gynecology patients and students of Vietnamese descent may have more difficulty with some Vietnam War veterans.

Finally, because many patients are distracted, confused, or hearing impaired, they may misunderstand what you would like to do. Patients have refused because they thought medical students wanted to give them a written test ("examine"), take them to surgery, give them an enema, change their bed sheets, take away their dinner plate, give them medications, switch their rooms, or change their bandages. Remember, many hospitalized patients see a constant stream of physicians, nurses, physical therapists, hospital representatives, phlebotomists, and technologists. It can be difficult for them to keep track of who does what.

Ultimately, because patients are under no obligation to permit medical students to talk to or examine them, it's their prerogative to refuse at any moment. Fortunately, for medical education, there are plenty of patients willing to help students.

What To Do

Don't take the refusal personally. Even if the patient is clearly biased against you, realize that the patient doesn't know you at all and her judgment may be impaired by illness or ignorance. Remain polite, thank the patient for her time, and leave the room. If you suspect that the patient is misunderstanding your request, you may politely ask again, explaining more carefully who you are and what you plan to do.

Remember, there will be plenty of other patients for you to examine, so finding another patient should be no problem. Don't let patient refusals affect your confidence. Be honest with your instructor. Because patient refusals happen all the time, it should in no way affect your grade or your instructor's impression of you.

Prevention and Preparation

If you find that many patients refuse your examination, perform an honest self-assessment. Consider asking friends to observe or videotape you. There are some things you can do to improve your chances of patients agreeing to your examination.

Come Clean

Make sure you and your clothes are clean. It will not only help you with patients, but potentially dramatically improve your social life.

Wearing Out Your Welcome

Patients may find certain articles of clothing and accessories too revealing or too off-beat. While wearing such items may express your individuality, an often important and worthwhile goal, unfortunately, it may also cost you patient acceptance. Ultimately, if you're wearing anything that patients may find unusual, you'll have to weigh the costs and benefits and decide whether it's worth dressing more conservatively for patient interviews.

Express Yourself . . . Appropriately

Patients may be disturbed, concerned, or even frightened by extreme expressions, such as those that make you look angry, bored, sad, or constipated. An appropriate smile can help, but excessive grinning like a Cheshire cat can make you appear disingenuous or slightly crazed. Be aware of what your eyes and body may be doing. Avoid rolling your eyes, finger tapping, winking, or any other movement that makes you look impatient or disdainful. Modulate your voice. Some students speak too softly, whereas others speak too loudly. Be careful about standing too close to or too far away from the patient.

Say What?

Be careful about what you say when you first meet the patient. Address the patient respectfully. It's safer to use appropriate titles, such as Mr., Mrs., or Ms., with the patient's last name rather than the patient's first name. Clearly introduce yourself and explain what you would like to do.

Timing Is Everything

Finally, don't choose times during which the patient is more likely to refuse an examination, such as when she's sleeping, meeting with visitors, eating, or sitting on the toilet. If you see that the patient is busy, consider returning when the patient is more available. After all, how would you feel if you were sitting on the toilet and someone walked in wanting to interview you?

What if . . .

Your patient doesn't speak English?

You walk into the patient's room, introduce yourself, explain that you'll be interviewing and doing a physical examination on the patient, and are met with a blank stare. The patient couldn't understand a single word you said because she doesn't speak English. What she heard was, "blah blah blah....blah." What do you do? Raising your voice when speaking ("BLAH, BLAH"), adding sounds "oh" and "ah" to the ends of the words ("blah-oh"), talking more slowly ("blaaaaaah...blaaaaah"), or repeating the words over and over ("blah?...blah?") won't help. Most physicians and medical students realize that non-English speakers aren't infants (unless, of course, they *are* infants), hard of hearing, or inattentive. Even so, for some reason, they commonly act as if altering the way of saying something will make a difference in their ability to communicate with the patient.

Such a situation is common; physicians often encounter immigrants, U.S. citizens living in communities that speak only foreign languages, and international travelers. Language barriers that may be easily surmountable when you're searching for a bathroom or ordering a meal can be devastating when providing medical care. Accidentally relaying the wrong diagnosis or instructions can be harmful and even deadly.

Please Pass the Sphygmomanometer?

Some physicians can speak other languages. However, being able to communicate in social situations doesn't guarantee that you can communicate in medical situations describing diseases, body parts, functions, symptoms, and treatments. Think about how hard it might be to describe a pneumothorax with limited vocabulary:

Physician: Ma'am, you have air in your lungs.

Patient: OK. That is good.

Physician: No, you don't understand. In addition to the air you are supposed to have in your lungs, you have air where you are not supposed to have air.

Patient: So I am breathing too much?

Word choice, intonations, and pronunciations can be important and complicated. Words that are synonyms according to a dictionary may have very different meanings. For example, if you had a growth on your foot, would you want a physician to "remove it," "amputate it," "rip it out," or "dismiss it"? Which statement would frighten you? Which would make you think the physician isn't going to do anything? Which would make you think the physician will be taking more than you anticipated? Consider the differences among words that sound the same or are spelled similarly, such as *bore, boar,* and *boor.* Would you rather have a *desert* or a *dessert?* In addition, understanding one dialect doesn't mean you can communicate in another dialect.

How Do You Say "Polite" in Spanish?

Sometimes it isn't obvious that the patient can't speak English. She may nod in agreement or appear to respond appropriately when she has no idea what you're saying. The patient may be acting politely, waiting for someone to talk to her in her language, suffering from delirium, or even mocking you. Appearances also can be deceiving. Never assume that a patient can or can't speak English and risk insulting or confusing her.

What To Do

First, if there is any doubt, confirm whether the patient can speak English. Don't accept simple nonverbal affirmation, such as head nodding and smiling. Give the patient an opportunity to respond verbally, if possible. Even if she can understand English, determine her speaking and comprehension level.

If the patient can't speak or understand English adequately, figure out what languages she can speak. The patient's name, place of residence, family members, friends, medical records, and possessions (such as books and identification cards) can provide clues, but beware of jumping to conclusions. Don't assume that a patient with the last name Martinez can speak Spanish or the last name Kim can speak Korean or someone with a home address in Athens, Greece, can speak Greek. If no definitive clues are available, try using different languages to see which ones the patient understands.

If possible, you'll need someone who can accurately communicate medical information in the languages spoken by the patient. If you aren't confident in your language skills, seek help. Official clinic or hospital translators are the best options, followed by fluent coworkers. If neither is available, the patient's family and friends may be able to translate.

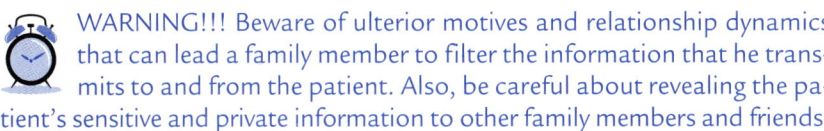

WARNING!!! Beware of ulterior motives and relationship dynamics that can lead a family member to filter the information that he transmits to and from the patient. Also, be careful about revealing the patient's sensitive and private information to other family members and friends.

If there isn't time or opportunity to find a translator, your only recourse may be to communicate visually, using pictures and gestures. Keep the concepts simple and straightforward and make sure you confirm as best as possible that the patient understands.

Prevention and Preparation

During your spare time, consider studying other languages. Even learning simple medical commands helps. Many medical schools and hospitals offer classes in Spanish for health-care settings. Typing "Medical Spanish" into a bookseller's website returns a list of dozens of books and software choices. Courses and instructional materials on other languages may be more difficult to find. If you can't find appropriate materials on websites, contact your medical school or hospital's education office for help to find the right course.

Being able to speak other languages could make you more marketable as a physician, especially if you want a job in places that have a wide range of ethnic groups such as California, New York City, and Florida. In general, the more experience you have interacting with people who are from other cultures and speak other languages, the more comfortable you'll be in this kind of situation. Know in advance how to reach translators in your hospital or clinic. Before you go in to see a patient, get a sense of what languages she speaks by reading the patient's chart and talking to people who have already seen the patient. If you prepare in this way, the patient won't have to ask herself, "What if I can't understand what my doctor is saying?"

What if . . .

Your patient is violent?

How safe are you in the hospital and the clinic? Many physicians and physicians-to-be are worried about walking home through "bad" neighborhoods, but fail to recognize the dangers that they face every day at work. They see patients with histories of violence, emotional disturbances, and psychiatric problems who are stressed by illness and the medical environment; these conditions are ingredients for violence. Did you know that, according to a study published in October 2003 by the British Medical Association's Health Policy and Economic Research Unit, more than one third of physicians had experienced violence from patients? Unruly behavior is a lot more commonplace in the hospital and clinic than in other workplace settings. Imagine what would happen if a client or customer started swinging his arms, spitting, or throwing things in a law firm, investment bank, or department store.

Physicians have been hurt badly and even killed by patients. The assaults can be accidental, deliberate, or even premeditated. Physicians can be innocent bystanders, targeted by their patients, or even randomly selected by people they don't know. In 1993, a man angry about people "diluting the Aryan beauty" murdered a plastic surgeon who he had randomly picked out of a phone book. Violent patients can not only inflict immediate physical harm, but also transmit dangerous infectious diseases such as HIV, hepatitis, and tuberculosis and cause significant psychological and emotional damage to their victims.

What To Do

If your patient becomes agitated, immediately leave the room, close the door, and call for security. No matter how many martial arts movies you've watched or how many siblings you have, you don't have the experience or ability to restrain the patient yourself. As soon as the patient intimates or threatens violence in any way, get help immediately. If you can't escape the room, yell or use the phone to call for help. Keep as much distance between you and the patient as possible.

Formally report all acts of violence. The British Medical Association study mentioned previously found that many victims had not reported acts of violence in the past. Reporting violence will help the hospital or clinic take steps to prevent future incidents by contacting the police, investing more in security, channeling such patients for appropriate psychiatric and behavioral health care and, perhaps, banning the patient from your clinic or hospital.

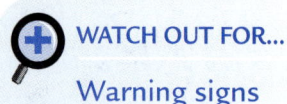

WATCH OUT FOR...

Warning signs

Always *subtly* assess a patient's risk of violence. (Of course, don't ask a patient if he "plans to kick your butt.") Be wary of patients who:

- have a history of violence against anyone.
- make inappropriate (sexual, racial, or unusually personal) comments.
- exhibit unpredictable, irrational, or inappropriate behavior.
- have significant emotional and personal problems.

Prevention and Preparation

Quickly assess all patients for their risk of violence. All patients, with the possible exception of newborns, can injure you. Never see a patient without potential help nearby. Only see high-risk patients when you're accompanied by psychiatric personnel or security guards. Patients who may harm themselves or anyone else may need to be restrained.

Have security guards disarm any patient carrying a firearm or other weapon. Don't try to disarm the patient yourself. Promptly remove or secure any items that may be used as weapons, such as unnecessary needles, blades, scalpels, and other sharp or bloody objects, such as IV lines, catheters, and orthopedic equipment. High-risk patients shouldn't be allowed to use metal utensils. Avoid wearing around your neck a stethoscope, loose necklaces, or anything else that may

- exhibit excessive dissatisfaction with waiting times, administrative hassles, medical care, and any other aspects of their clinic or hospital experience.
- carry weapons.
- have a history of significant psychiatric illness.
- are intoxicated or impaired by alcohol or drugs.
- seek controlled substances (as they may get violent when denied such substances).
- verbally abuse you or any of your colleagues.
- make any kind of threat, even in "jest."

be used to strangle you. Always be close to an unlocked, unobstructed exit. Never let the patient get between you and the exit. Know where security guards, telephones, fire alarms, and other colleagues are located at all times.

If your workplace doesn't have adequate security features (such as security guards, metal detectors, and escape routes), notify the hospital or clinic director. Don't wait for others to recognize the deficiencies; it may be too late.

Never argue with patients. Enlist the aid of properly trained personnel to handle disgruntled or agitated patients. Check with the clinic's front office or the hospital ward's nursing station to locate these specialists. When talking to patients, avoid controversial subjects. Disputes over sports teams, politics, and romantic interests have incited many fights and episodes of the Jerry Springer show. Remember, you're there to deal with the patient's medical problem, not indoctrinate the patient with your opinions.

Finally, have zero tolerance for violence. Report *all* situations that led to or may have led to violence. Don't tolerate even minor acts that cause no harm because minor acts can easily escalate to major acts. Remember, the hospital and clinic are your neighborhood, too. Try to keep it safe.

What if . . .

You have to assist in an operation you've never seen before?

In order to learn a tennis stroke or baseball swing, you must first visualize yourself doing each and every step of the motion. The better you can picture every detail, from positioning yourself, to striking the ball, to following through with your entire body, the better you'll perform when you actually have to complete the task.

Similarly, visualizing a medical procedure is the next best thing to doing it. The better you can visualize the procedure, the better you'll perform that first time, regardless of the circumstances. Conditions may not be ideal the first time you have to assist in an operation. The surgeon may be a poor teacher, impatient, in a hurry, or in a sour mood. Moreover, although no one will expect you to be skilled in the procedure the first time, being enthusiastic and knowledgeable about the procedure will certainly help earn you high marks.

What To Do

Adequately prepare so that you can visualize the operation. Once you are in the operating room, stay alert. Be friendly, respectful, and helpful to the surgical nurses, who can be very important allies and will commonly whisper advice to and subtly help students they like. Help lift the patient onto the operating room table and sterilize the incision site.

It's unlikely that a surgeon will require you to do anything technically difficult. Most likely you'll be holding and supporting things, doing your best impression of a mannequin. You'll be expected to hold clamps and retractors for very long periods of time firmly and still. Assisting in an operation can require significant physical and mental stamina, as some operations can last for hours. Avoid shaking, moving the clamps, falling asleep, drooling, or dropping things like your glasses into the surgical field. Frankly, watching someone operate for hours while you hold on for dear life to the retractor can be extremely dull. So you'll have to do your best to remain alert, focused, and ready to change positions or answer questions at a moment's notice.

If the surgeon allows you to cut or suture tissue, do so calmly and carefully. Confirm with the surgeon exactly where she wants the incision or stitch before commencing.

Prevention and Preparation

So how do you prepare? First understand the local anatomy that you'll encounter. For example, if you'll be assisting an appendectomy, know every blood vessel, muscle, organ, and tissue that surrounds the appendix. Find a good anatomical atlas with lots of pictures to help you visualize the anatomical landscape. Also, study the procedure. Read about the procedure in a surgical textbook. Look at the pictures that show how you should position your hands to hold retractors and clamps.

Know the disease being treated. For instance, for an appendectomy, know the incidence, causes, complications, symptoms, diagnostic testing, indications for surgery, treatment, and outcomes of appendicitis. Most surgical textbooks will have this information. Also, use MEDLINE to find a good review article on the subject. Several books provide answers to questions you're likely to be asked during each type of operation.

If possible, get to know the patient's medical problems, history, symptoms, and body size and shape by interviewing the patient and reading the chart. This knowledge will help you prepare for potential questions and better visualize the operation. Practice suturing and tying knots. Ask the surgical residents or nurses for a piece of surgical suture string, and practice suturing on a piece of cloth or meat, such as a pig's ear.

WARNING!!! Don't try to impress the surgeon with your technical skills so much that you end up making a mistake. Remember, the surgeon isn't evaluating you on your technical skill, but your enthusiasm, knowledge, and ability to work on a team.

Rest and get a good night's sleep. Wear comfortable (and appropriate) shoes. Go to the bathroom before the procedure. Don't eat anything that may give you diarrhea, an upset stomach, or flatulence. Remember, you'll be working in close quarters for hours, so make sure your bodily functions don't interfere. Otherwise, while visualizing the procedure, you may end up doing something that you definitely *don't* want to visualize.

What if . . .

Your family member is diagnosed with cancer at your own facility?

Shock, denial, anger, anxiety, sadness, fear, or confusion? How will you react when someone close to you becomes ill? No matter how composed and even-tempered you normally are, your emotions can become like a BMW without a steering wheel on a track coated with butter: unpredictable and uncontrollable. Sometimes, the strangest and seemingly most trivial things, such as hearing that song, seeing that floppy hat, or smelling the foot powder that you associate with your loved one, can trigger a torrent of emotions. At times, you may feel like a very bad soap opera actor, bawling, laughing, or seething at inappropriate times. And your work can easily suffer. Suddenly your mind is elsewhere. Grades, coursework, and tests may not seem so important anymore.

Are these signs of weakness or incompetence? No, they're signs that you're human. Because many people in medicine (and other high-achieving professions) are used to being in control of themselves and their situations, this apparent lack of control can be very disconcerting. However, there is no correct way to react. Emotional wounds are like bad physical wounds. Their damage can be hidden and deep and their course unpredictable. They'll hurt, need time to heal and, without proper management, have potentially serious consequences. (What's worse, emotional wounds don't respond at all to antibiotics.)

What To Do

Take care of yourself. Your family member will need you to be strong and healthy. Eat well, get enough sleep and exercise, and take time to relax. Although you may feel guilty about doing anything fun, forcing yourself to take occasional breaks to escape the pressure will help you better handle the situation. Seriously consider taking time off from school or work to rest and be there for your loved one. Your colleagues, instructors, and supervisors should understand. Don't take this the wrong way, but you're easily replaceable—especially because your work quality will likely suffer.

Express Yourself

Don't be too hard on yourself and expect normal functioning. Acknowledge and express your emotions and feelings. Allow yourself to cry and get angry, among other emotions. Expect memory and concentration lapses.

No Man or Woman Is an Island

Don't be an island (unless it's Hawaii, which might be fun). Allow yourself to be helped by your supervisors, colleagues, and friends. Consider yourself fortunate if you have people who care for you and want to help. Don't let pride or concerns about your "image" prevent you from seeking support. Many challenges are too tough to face alone.

Choose Your Team and Let Them Do What They Do Best

Your "inside" knowledge of your medical center and the reputations, personalities, and expertise of its people can help your loved one find the right physicians and help navigate through the bureaucratic maze. Once you've helped choose the right physicians, though, try not to interfere with their care. Your lack of experience and objectivity can be dangerous. Many coaches say that the key to coaching is selecting the right players and then getting out of the way and letting them play. Similarly, although you certainly should feel free to ask questions, offer your help, and keep abreast of what is happening, learn to relinquish control. Allow the chosen experts to do what they do best, and permit them to run the show.

Cutting the Grapevine

Medical centers can be fishbowls with active gossip mills. Your colleagues and the team caring for your loved one should respect your right to privacy and confidentiality. If your colleagues become too nosy, gently remind them that it's none of their business and ask them how they would feel if your roles were reversed. If the health-care team accidentally leaks information, remind them of their obligation to you and your loved one.

Difficult People

Some colleagues and supervisors may have never experienced misfortune, not understand your situation and needs, and, as a result, be tactless, inappropriate, and even difficult. Unfortunately, some may even deliberately try to take advantage of your misfortune, such as using it as an opportunity to get a better grade or evaluation than you. Although these people must realize "what goes around comes around," in such a situation, the last thing you need is to spend valuable time and energy arguing with and trying to change the mindset of these closed-minded individuals. Get a reasonable third party (such as the course director, medical school dean of students, or ombudsperson) involved as quickly as possible.

Prevention and Preparation

Take time to develop and maintain relationships with your family, friends, and colleagues. Don't sacrifice the social and familial aspects of your life. (Come on, is getting that higher test score and class ranking really worth it?) Many physicians remember very little from medical school coursework or board exam studying. (The first year of medical school teaches you something about splicing or wearing genes.) However, they cherish the friendships they developed and the time they spent with loved ones. Having a network of dependable people can provide not only enjoyment, more players for pick-up basketball games, and better dinner parties, but also valuable support when hard times come.

Don't wait until bad times to look for supportive friends. If you've spent years insulting, competing with, and offending others, you may find few people willing to help you. In addition, people who don't seem cool or power-ful enough for you may in fact be your most valuable friends in the future. Consider building relationships to be an investment in yourself because, when your BMW loses it steering wheel, it's great to know that you have a bunch of Yugos, Metros, Neons, Hyundais, and Prisms around you to guide you down the track.

Notes

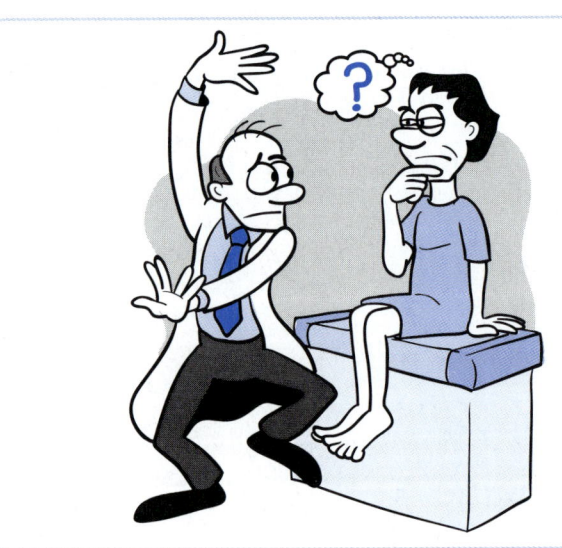

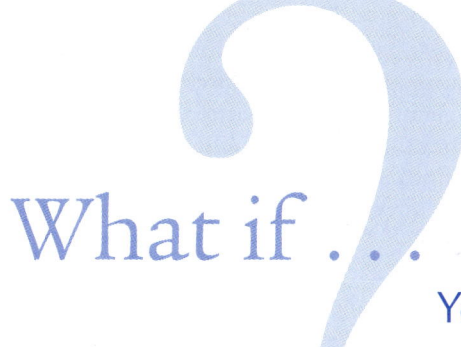

What if . . .

You're examining your first deaf patient?

Deaf patients are commonly misunderstood. Because they may focus on a person's lips to lip-read or hands to read sign language, they don't always maintain eye contact during conversations. They may not be able to detect or use the different tones of voice, inflections, and timely pauses that many people use to communicate. When amongst a group of people, a deaf patient will usually pay greatest attention to the person using sign language, rather than the person speaking or the one with the highest rank. As a result, consciously or unconsciously, people may feel put off or even offended by the deaf patient.

It's remarkable how much we rely on subtle expressions, positioning, and voice to interpret what someone is saying and to form an opinion about the person, which, unfortunately, puts deaf patients at a disadvantage. So when you encounter a deaf patient for the first time, realize that his or her facial expressions, body positioning, and reactions may be different from what you're accustomed to. Realize, though, that like anyone from a different "culture," deaf patients beneath the surface are no different from other patients. They have the same diversity of backgrounds, experiences, abilities, and problems that all patients have.

What To Do

Gather as much information as possible before the interview to minimize the amount that you need to collect during the interview. Carefully read the patient's medical record and consider giving the patient written medical history questionnaires beforehand. Check with the hospital or clinic front desk, nursing station, or telephone operator to find out if interpretation services are available. Many hospitals and clinics have interpreters fluent in sign language or telecommunication devices for the deaf.

To find the appropriate interpreter, you may have to determine what type of manual language the patient prefers. The most common is American Sign Language (ASL), which isn't visualized English, but a distinctly different language. Pidgin Signed English (PSE) also uses signs but has syntax closer to English. Finger spelling and Signing Exact English (SEE) use hands to spell out English words. Sometimes patients and their families have developed their own variations of sign language.

Never force a deaf patient to talk. Also, never assume or insist that the patient lip-reads. Similarly, never assume that the patient knows or wants to communicate in a certain type of sign language. Not allowing the patient to use the form of communication that he feels most comfortable using can insult and alienate the patient.

Be patient when working with a sign-language interpreter for the first time. The interpreter has to first understand what you're trying to say before she starts signing to the patient and may not know the signs needed to communicate certain medical terms and concepts. The interpreter's and the patient's speed, comprehension, vocabulary, and fluency can vary significantly. Therefore, give them ample opportunity and time to become acquainted with each other and correctly communicate. Allow the interpreter to drive the pace of the interview.

If no formal interpreters are available, then use alternative methods of communication. One method is spelling out your words on a piece of paper or computer in large, clear letters. Because some patients aren't used to English syntax, include only key words and exclude articles and other unnecessary modifiers. Alternatively, many patients can lip-read. When talking, face the patient, speak slowly, and make sure that your face is well-lit. Whenever possible, use simpler words instead of medical terminology.

Prevention and Preparation

Interviewing and examining a deaf patient will commonly require additional time and planning. Allot enough time on your schedule and request the necessary medical records in advance. Know where to go for interpretation services and inform them about your patient as early as possible so that they can reserve the appropriate interpreter. The more you work with deaf patients, the more comfortable you'll be. So don't wait until you're assigned a deaf patient. Contact your medical school or medical center's otology division (usually part of the otolaryngology, ENT, or head and neck department) to get resources and, possibly, more experience. Working with deaf patients can teach you a lot about people and yourself. Remember, we commonly put far too much stock in voice, appearance, body positioning, and expressions when forming our judgments. There is usually much more to a person than you may first see . . . or hear.

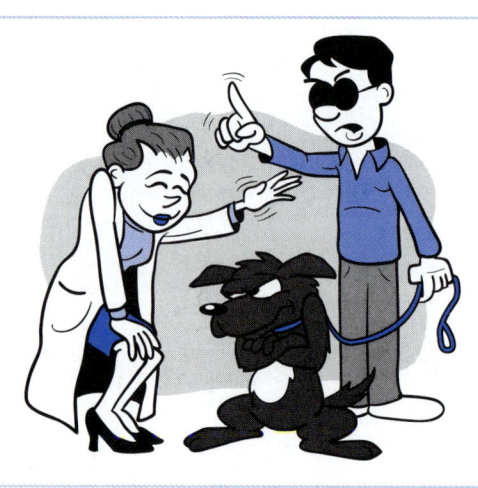

What if . . .

You're examining your first blind patient?

Think about how much visual information you process every day. When you first meet someone, you examine the person's face, facial expressions, body positioning, posture, body size and shape, clothing, uniform, and identification badge, forming impressions immediately. A room's location, lighting, size, shape, and furniture affect where you move, how you act, and what to expect. Visual cues can help you anticipate future actions and events. For example, someone with a mop is likely to clean your room and someone carrying syringes and needles may be looking to draw blood. If visual information didn't play such an important role in our society, Heidi Klum, Giorgio Armani, and Andy Warhol may not have made the money they did.

Patients who are unable to collect visual information have to rely on other senses. When you enter a visually impaired patient's room without proper introduction, the patient doesn't know who you are and whether you're there to provide food, mop the floor, or perform a rectal examination—or all three. Needless to say, such an ambush could be very disconcerting.

What To Do

Introduce yourself as soon as you enter the room and clearly identify your function and the reason you're there. Be careful about startling the patient. Know and confirm the patient's level of visual disability so that you may appropriately tailor your interaction. If, for example, only the patient's peripheral vision is impaired, then you simply have to make sure you stay in the patient's field of vision. Make anyone who walks into the room aware of the nature and degree of the patient's visual disability in an appropriate manner. Remember, a person is much more than her visual disability and should never be defined by it. So never refer to a patient as "the blind woman."

Can't Touch This

Don't touch or move mobility canes unless the patient asks you to do so. If you move anything, specify exactly where you're moving it. Moving even seemingly insignificant objects may disrupt the landscape and confuse the patient. Hand objects to the patient, rather than leaving them next to the patient. Dog guides should be allowed in hospitals and health-care facilities, unless their presence somehow endangers or jeopardizes other people or safe operations. Don't feed, pet, distract, or move dog guides. Only the owner should control the dog guide.

Being There

Offer but never impose assistance. The patient may ask you to read menus, consent forms, bills, advance directive forms, medication labels, or other documents. If the document contains financial or medical information, to preserve confidentiality, make sure no one else is around. If the documents are extensive or may need to be reviewed by the patient in the future, offer to find Braille, large print, or taped versions, which hospitals commonly have. The patient also may need help completing menus, identifying items on the meal tray, positioning food on the tray, or cutting meat.

Talk the Talk Before Walking the Walk

If the patient needs assistance standing up or walking, offer your arm and allow the patient to hold onto it for support. Don't actively grab, push, or pull the patient. Walk at a relaxed, normal pace with the patient a step or two behind you. Warn the patient of any changes in direction or terrain and don't proceed until the patient has acknowledged your warning. When the patient needs to sit down, offer to show him or her the back of the chair and, if the patient wants you to, guide the patient's hand to touch the chair back.

When giving directions, be very specific. Right and left should be from the patient's perspective, not yours. Whenever you can, provide exact numbers—for example, "The door is 10 feet away," or "The room is 7 doors down the hallway." Provide as much relevant detail as possible. When a patient enters a new room, offer the patient a walk-around orientation. Clearly describe any procedures or physical examination techniques that you plan to perform. Let the patient touch and inspect any equipment that you'll be using. Unless the patient is hard of hearing, there is no need to raise your voice. Aside from being sensitive to the patient's needs, you should talk as you would normally talk to other patients. Face and talk directly to the patient. When you're ready to leave, tell the patient, otherwise she may not realize that you've left.

Prevention and Preparation

Get into the habit of evaluating a patient's vision because the patient's visual impairment may not yet be diagnosed or documented. Some patients don't notice or won't admit vision problems, which ultimately can endanger them when they're driving, taking medications, or performing other daily activities.

Practice verbally describing different procedures and parts of the physical examination. It may not be as easy as it initially seems because we do many things unconsciously and generally take visual information for granted. Television, movies, and advertising have made our society increasingly visual to the point that we typically can't see beyond what we can see. So, practicing how to use and communicate through other senses can have benefits beyond your clinical experience.

What if . . .

You're being one-upped by another student during rounds?

Highly competitive medical students—you have observed them, worked with them, or have had them work for you. Or perhaps you're one of them. (If you are, stop one-upping other students!) Unfortunately, not everyone realizes that in the long run, blind competition will hurt more than help a career. In medicine, you have to work with a wide variety of people and unless you're able to do so harmoniously and productively, you may face endless hassles at every stage of your career. (Also, few people will want to eat dinner with you, but that's another *What if.*)

Not all medical students realize how they're evaluated. Showing off that you have memorized *Harrison's Principles of Medicine* may get you a spot on a game show such as *Jeopardy,* but that alone won't earn you better grades. Attendings and residents are looking to see how well you work in a team. Therefore, trying to make your fellow medical students look bad is very risky, not advisable (and, of course, not very nice). Remember, there are few things worse to have on an evaluation than "not a team player" or "lacks social skills."

So, how may other medical students one-up you and try to make you look bad during rounds? They may try to demonstrate that they know more about your patients than you do, highlight your shortcomings, or put you in difficult situations. They may withhold important information from the attending that they should relay to you. In severe cases, they may try to directly sabotage your work.

What To Do

Calling the other medical student names (unless you can think of some very clever names) will make you look infantile, and *infantile* is another word you don't want on your evaluation. Trying to one-up the one-upper is similar to an escalating nuclear arms race, both sides are likely to end up losing.

The first time someone does it to you, maintain your composure and don't act flustered. Perhaps it's a one-time occurrence and will have little effect on anything. Perhaps no one else noticed. If you overreact, it may actually adversely affect you. In sports, they say that fouls are usually called on the retaliator and not the person who initiated the fight because referees commonly miss the initial blow. It isn't fair, but it's reality.

If the one-upper one-ups you more than once, first determine the effect that the one-upping is having. Many attendings and residents have enough experience to detect (and typically detest) the games that some medical students play. If they do realize what is happening, the one-upper may be doing you a favor, making himself or herself look bad and you look better by comparison. In this case, just relax, smile, and concentrate on the people that you can control—such as yourself.

If you feel that the higher-ups are being influenced by or encouraging this behavior (sadly, some do), then you may have to take action. Tell the other student in private what you think about his actions. There is a chance that the other student's actions are unintentional. Don't be confrontational but be firm. Convince him that cooperation will make both of you look better. No one says that you can't both get high grades.

If the other student is still uncooperative, the final resort is a frank conversation with the

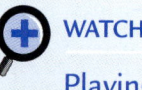

WATCH OUT FOR...

Playing the game

Caution! You may decide to play the game. Playing the game means going into the hospital around 6 o'clock in the morning to chat with the night nurses and learn about the admissions that came in during the night. Then a quick review of your resources (such as the library or Internet), puts you "in the know." You can propose brilliant differential diagnoses. You'll quote the most recent research and you can even cite specific references! Before you know it, you're the number-one one-upper!!! Don't fall into this trap. Simply be well prepared.

attending. Rather than impugn the other student's character, simply relay what you feel about the other student's actions. Remember you don't want to turn this into a mudslinging competition. Stick to the facts. For example, rather than saying that the other student is cutthroat and devious, tell the attending that it bothers you when the other student points out your mistakes during rounds. Emphasize that your goal isn't to criticize the other student, but instead curtail the other student's actions. Again, there is a good chance the attending already understands the situation. If not, then you have alerted the attending to the problem.

Prevention and Preparation

At the beginning of a class or rotation, the attending can set the tone by announcing to everyone her expectations. If the attending emphasizes teamwork and fair play and frowns on competitiveness, the potential one-uppers may realize that they won't gain anything by cutthroat behavior. Although it's reasonable to ask the attending to review her expectations to everyone, it's certainly up to the attending to decide what tone she wants to set.

Work hard to improve yourself. The more the attending is impressed by you, the less likely she'll be to be affected by the one-upper. Develop good relationships with everyone else on the team. If you get along with everyone else, the one-upper's actions will appear more unwarranted by comparison. Do what you can to avoid and mitigate potential one-upping situations. If you know the other student will try to highlight your shortcomings during rounds, be prepared and know your patients. If the other student is withholding important information from you, then be extra vigilant about what you need to know. Naturally, if you have to choose between working with the one-upper and other students, choose the other students.

If all of this fails, keep things in perspective. In your career, you'll continue to run into people who don't play fair. Sometimes they'll get away with it and even thrive at your expense. But in the long run, staying above it will yield greater benefits. Realize that one rotation won't make or break your career. Think of this situation as practice for life—something far more important than a single medical school rotation.

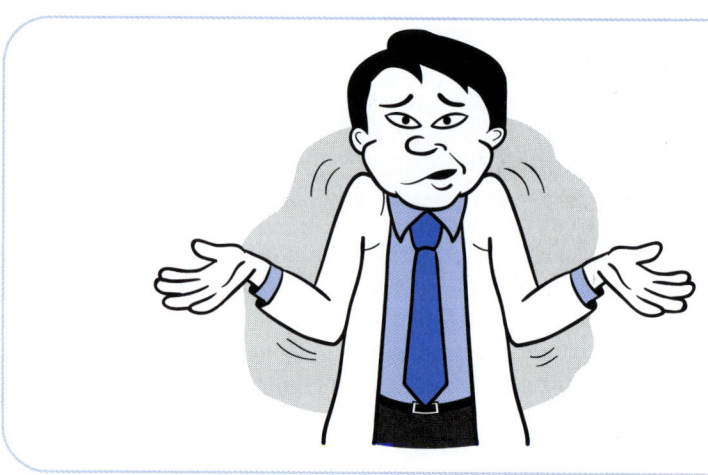

What if . . . You're asked by a senior clinician, "Have you ever seen one of these done before"?

"It's my first time." Maybe these aren't the words you want to utter on a first date. But how about in a medical school rotation or class when the senior clinician asks how many times you've seen a certain procedure performed? Are you worried about appearing naïve or inexperienced? This may be your one and only chance to impress someone who you feel is very important. After all, who's going to notice if you tell an itty-bitty white lie and claim that you have more experience than you actually have?

You may say that poker players bluff all the time and advertisers, entertainers, job seekers, politicians, and lawyers commonly exaggerate the benefits of their products or their own attributes. However, in this situation, what are the potential benefits and dangers of not being straightforward about your experience?

The only potential benefit is impressing the clinician. However, because most clinicians have seen so many medical students, house staff, and other physicians, the clinician probably won't be impressed by the number of procedures you claim to have done. Moreover, quantity doesn't necessarily equal quality. Having done a procedure many times doesn't guarantee that you're adept at the procedure.

What are the dangers? The clinician may make you prove your claim by quizzing you or having you perform the procedure in front of everyone. Then, if you appear nervous, perform poorly, or require significant help, you'll look incompetent instead of simply inexperienced. Worse, you could seriously injure the patient.

So, what about the opposite approach: being straightforward about your experience (or inexperience)? If you're honest, the clinician may take extra time and effort to teach you the procedure, an excellent opportunity to learn and have quality contact with the clinician. You can impress him with your enthusiasm, attitude, and learning ability. In fact, setting low expectations will make it easier for you to impress him. For example, successfully completing a procedure on your first attempt will make you look like "a natural" and "a quick learner" and the clinician look like a good teacher.

What To Do

Be straightforward about your experience. However, emphasize that you would relish the opportunity to learn from the clinician. In the world of medical evaluations, enthusiasm (and a little flattery) easily overshadows inexperience. Don't be defensive if the clinician asks you why you haven't seen the procedure. Simply, respond that you haven't yet had the opportunity. Reasonable physicians realize that getting appropriate experience in the hospital can be difficult. Blaming previous teachers or finding excuses will make you look petty and disingenuous.

Err on the side of underselling your previous experience. Don't count previous experi-

WATCH OUT FOR...

Watching and not doing

Don't get stuck in the "watch-one-more" rut! Yes, it's good to watch a procedure performed before you try it with an instructor. However, watching it done multiple times before attempting it will not only not help you, but may prevent you from ever getting the chance to do it. There is nothing as good as "hands-on learning." Your clinical rotations consist of a fair amount of serendipitous opportunities to learn and do. You need to grab those opportunities. If a thoracic surgeon offers to show you how to do an emergency tracheostomy, wash your hands and put on some sterile gloves. She isn't going to let you hurt the patient. You can't watch or read about the feeling you get through the needle when that needle pops into place during a lumbar puncture. You have to feel it!

The old adage, "Watch one, do one, teach one," may be an exaggeration, but perhaps only in the "teach one" part of the phrase.

ences that you feel were inadequate. (Maybe you only saw part of the procedure or weren't taught well.)

Prevention and Preparation

During medical school and training, you'll have dozens and dozens of different teachers, each of whom is swamped by clinical, research, teaching, administrative, and personal responsibilities. Outstanding teachers with enough time are hard to find. No one will keep track of what you have properly learned. So it's commonly your responsibility to get proper teaching and experience. The further you go along in your career, the harder it is to admit that you haven't learned something. Be proactive and take every opportunity to learn a procedure. Don't wait for the opportunity to learn something. Find and ask good teachers to teach you.

While no one can blame you for a lack of experience, they can blame you for a lack of effort. Even on a first date, admitting that it's your first time may not be such a bad thing. Your date may have a thing or two to teach you.

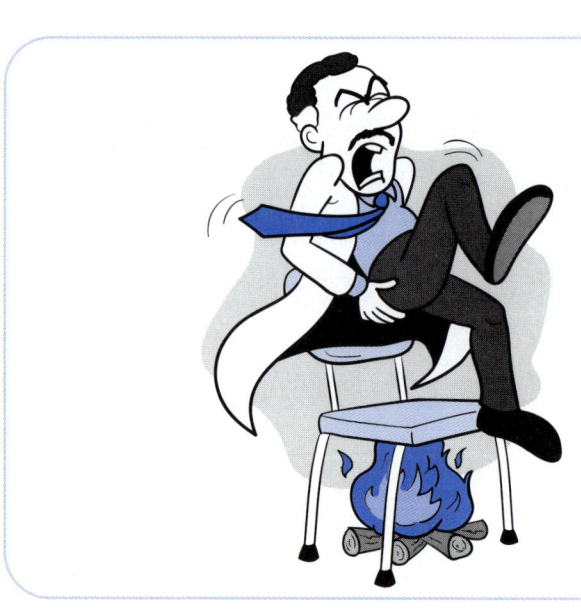

What if . . .

You're on the "hot seat" during morning rounds with a professor, attending physician, or other senior clinician?

It's amazing what can happen when someone is put on the "hot seat." The most outgoing and sociable students can lose the ability to talk. The most knowledgeable can forget answers to basic questions. The most poised can melt in a pool of sweat. Call it *stage fright, performance anxiety,* or *nerves,* funny things can happen when you feel exposed in front of a group of people.

Several things can happen when you're on the "hot seat." You can be asked any number or types of questions. The attending can be friendly or antagonistic, patient or impatient, attentive or distracted. You can be expected to give a presentation, perform a procedure, or interview and examine a patient. Sometimes people are placed on the "hot seat," only to have the entire time taken up by the attending talking. At any moment the "hot seat" may switch to another student. The length of time on the "hot seat" can vary significantly. A student can stay on the "hot seat" for the entire length of rounds, which can last for hours.

The ostensible purposes of the hot seat are to teach, communicate, and evaluate. By asking you questions, the attending can force you to think about and understand the material. Your answers will teach other medical students, house staff, and people in attendance. The "hot seat" can also be a way of transferring information about patients to the attending. However, the attending will also be developing an impression of you, especially if he or she has had little exposure to you. In some situations, it will be a busy attending's only time to evaluate you, which isn't fair but is reality, nevertheless. Of course, some attendings enjoy putting medical students on the "hot seat" and acting like a quizmaster or oracle or seeing students squirm. In some cases, the teaching and communication purposes of the "hot seat" can be lost.

How you perform on the "hot seat" is commonly not an accurate reflection of your knowledge and abilities. Some people actually appear better than they are. Many appear worse. In addition to your ability and experience in handling such a situation, a lot of luck is involved. Does the attending seem to be in a good mood, like you personally, or ask you questions in areas that are your strengths or weaknesses? Did you have adequate time to prepare? Sometimes being on the "hot seat" can be expected or unexpected. Are the setting and the people around you familiar?

What To Do

The best way to improve your performances on the "hot seat," is to gain experience. Find situations to give patient presentations and answer questions. Some of the best public speakers were nervous and awkward at some point in their lives. Even department chairpersons and hospital executives are regularly put on the "hot seat" by deans, physicians, students, boards of directors, and various committees.

Don't be afraid of saying you don't know or that you're guessing. Commonly, a student enters a spiral in which he makes guesses, the attending knows that he's guessing and presses harder, and the student makes additional, wilder guesses, and everyone in attendance starts squirming.

Do what you can to relax. Don't be intimidated by the attending. He or she is just a

 WATCH OUT FOR...

Analysis paralysis

If you're on the hot seat, you're under pressure and it's likely you'll have trouble remembering things you actually know. When asked the hot-seat question, your mind will go blank. Don't panic! Buy some time to think. Repeat the question out loud as if you're trying to make sure you've understood the question (because, in fact, you do need to understand the question).

Most questions on rounds are actually fairly simple and straightforward. No one is looking for a PhD thesis for an answer. Don't overanalyze the question. Don't suspect that it's a trick question. Don't presume the first simplistic answer that comes to your mind is wrong. It's probably the correct answer. When all else fails you, start talking about the things you know that may be related. The answer may reveal itself!

person and has been on the "hot seat" many times as well. Treat the situation like an opportunity to learn and gain experience rather than an evaluation.

Much of the other advice that applies to public speaking or interviewing applies to the "hot seat." Maintain eye contact, be aware of your body posture, smile when appropriate, speak clearly, and pause when appropriate. If someone corrects you, acknowledge their suggestions and don't appear defensive.

Prevention and Preparation

When the opportunity to be on the "hot seat" arises, don't decline, unless of course there is an obvious reason to do so, such as lack of preparation (or severe diarrhea). Otherwise, you'll forfeit an important opportunity to gain experience for the many times in the future when you'll be on the "hot seat" as a medical student, resident, and attending. To avoid forfeiting the "hot seat" opportunity, always be prepared—especially if you know that you'll be in such a situation. Know not only the material and your patients, but also the people who'll be putting you on the "hot seat." The more familiar the surroundings and people, the more comfortable you'll be. If for instance, you know that the attending tends to be rather gruff and grouchy, then you won't be taken aback when he or she acts that way.

Most of all, don't fret if you happen to do less than your best while on the "hot seat." There will be many other opportunities and, with each experience, that seat won't feel quite as hot.

I WILL NOT OFFEND A PATIENT
I WILL NOT OFFEND A PATIENT
I WILL NOT OFFEND A PATIENT
I WILL NOT OFFEND A PATIENT
I WILL NOT OFFEND A PATIENT
I WILL NOT OFFEND A
I WILL NO

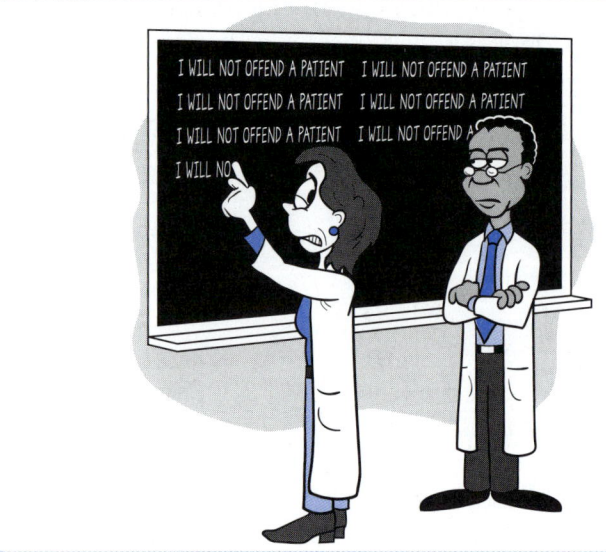

What if . . .

You feel the way that a colleague speaks to or about patients is inappropriate?

Although inappropriate comments may occur in any setting, the medical environment's stress, pressure, and unique emotional context make them even more likely to occur. These comments can be sexist or racist remarks, sexual comments, derogatory statements, and information on someone's personal situation, with patients, colleagues, or strangers being the targets.

Inappropriate comments don't have to be derogatory. Comments appropriate in some settings may be inappropriate in others. Patient confidentiality laws bolstered by the Health Insurance Portability and Accountability Act (HIPAA) outlaw the sharing of patient information beyond specific patient care and research reasons.

Never underestimate the potential damage. Comments can be hurtful, ruin reputations, create an atmosphere of distrust, and also lead to formal complaints, legal action, and dismissals. Just imagine people that you trust making derogatory statements about you or disclosing intimate details about your life.

Comments can be deliberate or unintentional, out of malice or just ignorance. There is really no good reason to make such comments. There are more mature, productive, creative, and effective ways to relieve stress, be funny, attract attention, or deal with people you dislike. Someone who criticizes or discredits others looks not only immature, but also petty.

What To Do

Of course, the situation is easier to handle if the comment was an accidental, one-time occurrence made out of ignorance rather than malice. A person with a history of making inappropriate comments may be more difficult to handle. Here are some general principles:

1. *Resolve the situation soon.* Before you say anything, give the person an opportunity to retract or apologize for the comment. However, don't wait too long; discuss the comment while details are still fresh and the damage can be minimized.
2. *Avoid discussing the situation in front of other people.* People are more likely to admit that they're wrong in private. If you need to, tell the person you have something important you want to discuss in private.
3. *Create a constructive atmosphere.* Putting people on the defensive makes them less likely to accept criticism. Therefore, don't attack the person or raise your voice. Critique the comment—not the person—and offer ways that he can make amends. For example, instead of saying, "You were offensive," say, "What you said may have offended the patient." Separating the comment from the person makes him more likely to view the comment objectively.
4. *Identify situations where help may be needed.* If the person is a repeat offender, is antagonistic, or threatens you, get help. Most schools and universities have ombudspersons who provide confidential guidance and assistance. Check your school's handbook to locate them. Using proper channels will protect you from retaliation.

Prevention and Preparation

Preventing inappropriate comments requires an understanding about why they're made. A majority of such comments come from ignorance or insecurity. Many people have lived rather insulated lives and have had only superficial or atypical contact with members of a group other than their own; therefore, they rely on stereotypes generated by the movies, television, friends, or family. They also may not realize how hurtful their comments can be. For these people, education works. Describe or introduce people who don't fit the stereotypes (which is easy, since most people don't actually match stereotypes). Also, reverse the situation: Ask them how they would feel if someone were to make similar inappropriate comments about them or their groups. Sometimes giving actual examples can be effective. Some people discount how offensive comments can be until they're the target. Remember, all of us stereotype to some degree. Every day is a chance to learn more about a group that we assume we already understood.

Comments arising from insecurity may be more difficult to prevent. People unhappy with their own situations may look for a scapegoat or someone to bully to make themselves feel better. They may view certain groups as "threats" and try to make preemptive strikes. Of course, the real solution is for them to improve their own lives (and stop worrying about other people) or accept the situation and give credit to other people. The key is convincing them to opt for one of these solutions. An older physician once complained that his department was being taken over by "stupid women and funny-looking minorities." We explained to him that many of the best people in his field happen to be women and mi-

 WATCH OUT FOR...

Laughter: Not the best medicine

He who laughs last doesn't know it's a joke! All too often physicians are tempted to show how cleverly humorous they can be. Don't become the problem! Our stressful work and our clever minds make us prone to making quips we think are funny (as a way to reduce stress) or even using sarcasm as humor. What's more, long, stressful hours of work can make us irritable and intolerant of patients' questions or their care-seeking behavior (such as an ER visit at 3 a.m. complaining of back pain that began 6 months ago).

Don't fall into this trap. Patients aren't seeking humor from you and don't expect you to be funny. Patients are worried and looking for answers and reassurance. A physician's clever remarks or attempts at humor aren't well-received and are commonly misinterpreted. You'll never get a patient to follow your instructions or take medications you prescribe if they think you're a "jokester."

Understand and remember that your patients haven't had the medical education and training that you have. When patients say things that don't make sense to you, there's probably a reason. It's probably a clue that you need to ask more questions and ferret out the reason for the strange answer. If the patient were looking for a laugh, they'd go to a comedy club, not the doctor!

norities and asked him if he would rather have less competent people around, which would create more work and hassle for him.

Signs, Signs, Everywhere Signs

There are signs that an inappropriate comment is about to be made, such as a pause, knowing glance, mischievous look, or wink. People will sometimes look like a kid about to raid the cookie jar. If you notice this behavior, nudge the person or interject with an unrelated question to suppress the impending comment. Sometimes conversations or situations can provide natural lead-ins to inappropriate comments (for example, a patient wondering out loud why he has contracted so many sexually transmitted diseases over the past year). If you notice such a lead-in, try to change the course of the conversation before anyone has a chance to speak. (For example, you could say, "Well, the reason why you contracted the diseases isn't important right now. What's important is treating it and getting you better.")

Get Educated

Many medical schools and medical centers have sensitivity training workshops and courses, designed to make people more aware about this problem. Convincing people to take these courses seriously may help them better handle such situations and realize the harm in comments they're making. After all, everyone has made inappropriate comments to some degree. If you don't believe you ever have, you should be looking more carefully, as we're all human and fallible. The difference is, some people recognize and admit when they've made such a mistake, feel truly contrite, and take measures to prevent it in the future.

Notes

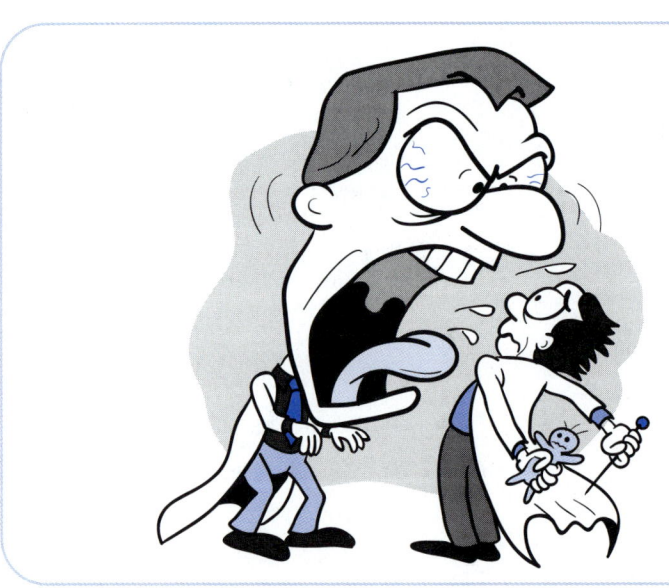

What if . . .

You're faced with a tyrannical colleague?

It's a prehistoric jungle out there. Like reality television show contestants, tyrannical colleagues *(Tyrannosaurus colleagi)* are everywhere. If you haven't encountered one, you're very lucky or you're *the* tyrannical colleague of your workplace. *Tyrannosaurus colleagi* can strike in many different ways, directly (such as openly abusing you verbally or physically), or indirectly (such as discrediting or hurting you behind your back), and in obvious or subtle ways. They can commit the acts themselves, assemble allies to help them, or use their trusted henchpeople or subordinates to carry out their dirty work. Some are so subtle, that you don't even realize that you have a tyrannical colleague.

What To Do

Of course, only you can decide whether you want to do anything about your tyrannical colleague. Many people quietly suffer for years under a *Tyrannosaurus colleagus* because they don't know what to do, fear the consequences of taking action, don't feel that it's worth the effort to change their situation, or are waiting for others to rescue them. However, many people don't realize the emotional, physical, and professional toll inflicted by a tyrannical colleague, until the tyrannical colleague is no longer in the workplace. Remember, unless you take action, your situation is unlikely to change. If you want to take action, then how you handle *Tyrannosaurus colleagi* depends on the species of *Tyrannosaurus.*

Socially Ineptasaurus

Description: Doesn't understand social customs and norms; is completely unaware that she's offensive and hurtful.

Possible Origin: Sheltered upbringing, social inexperience.

Signs: Irrational, counterproductive actions.

How to handle this species: In private, explain why her behavior is hurtful and not socially acceptable. Suggest alternative, healthier ways of dealing with people.

Emotionosaurus

Description: Can't control his emotions; inadvertently hurts colleagues in fits of anger.

Possible Origin: Lack of healthy emotional outlets.

Signs: Tyrannical acts are accompanied by seething, red faces, drooling, spitting, or general lack of control of bodily functions.

How to handle this species: Suggest safe, healthy outlets for anger, such as exercising, meditation, hobbies, and Brittany Spears concerts.

Power Hungrisaurus (or Megalomaniasaurus)

Description: Dictatorial and obsessed with power

Possible Origin: Deep-seated insecurity? Upbringing? Revenge?

Signs: Calculated and purposeful.

How to handle this species: This particular species can be difficult to handle. Avoid them, if possible. If you must interact with them, try to convince them that treating you terribly won't aid (and perhaps will even inhibit) their quest for power. Consider negotiating with them—for example, "If you treat me in a reasonable manner, I will complete the work as efficiently as possible." You may need help from an impartial person (such as an ombudsperson) or a more powerful person (such as the supervisor of the Power Hungrisaurus).

Temporary Tyrannosaurus

Description: Normally reasonable *(Reasonablesaurus),* but has suddenly turned tyrannical.

Possible Origin: A difficult life event (such as a relationship, family, or work problem) makes her edgy and irritable.

Signs: Normally stable but becomes suddenly emotionally labile.

How to handle this species: Realize that this is a temporary and unnatural state. If it isn't causing significant problems, consider "riding out the storm" until the Tyrannosaurus turns back into a Reasonablesaurus. Offer emotional support and help.

Scapegoatasaurus

Description: Abuses innocent colleagues and subordinates to release his own frustrations and insecurities.

Possible Origin: His own frustrations and insecurities.

Signs: May target and make broad sweeping generalizations about certain groups.

How to handle this species: Make it clear to the *Scapegoatasaurus* that he'll only make his own situations worse by alienating colleagues.

Revengesaurus

Description: Seeks revenge against you.

Possible Origin: Feeling, correctly or incorrectly, that you or a group you belong to (such as people of the same gender, race, country, age, social group, or political group as you) has wronged her; may be very similar to *Scapegoatasaurus.*

Signs: Deliberately tries to hurt, sabotage, or discredit you.

How to handle this species: Determine what you may have done to offend the *Revengesaurus* by reviewing your own actions and talking to her. If you indeed did something wrong, make amends. If you didn't, convince the *Revengesaurus* that you haven't done anything deliberately to harm her. If this fails, you may need help from an impartial or more powerful person.

Bullysaurus

Description: Just like the bully from grade school.

Possible Origin: History of being bullied himself by his superiors, parents, and others; inability to stand up against his own persecutors that leads to his bullying behavior toward others.

Signs: Enjoys belittling or humiliating you.

How to handle this species: Because a bully commonly fears anyone who stands up to him, stand up for yourself and make it clear that you won't be bullied. In all cases, if your initial attempts are unsuccessful, consider consulting your school or medical center's ombudsperson or equivalent.

Chemically Impairedasaurus

Description: Uncharacteristic destructive or unpredictable thoughts and actions while under the influence of substances or disease.

Possible Origin: Drugs, alcohol, medications, medical conditions, or withdrawal from drugs or alcohol that can affect her judgment and behavior.

Signs: History of substance abuse or illness.

How to handle this species: She needs appropriate professional help. If she's already under the care of professionals, be tolerant and understanding of her situation.

Prevention and Preparation

Stay alert. Don't be naïve and get blindsided by tyrannical colleagues. Sometimes *Tyrannosaurus colleagi* will test the waters by committing minor acts against you to see how you respond before they become bolder and more vicious. Allowing too many minor acts to occur without taking action may cause the situation to mushroom. Therefore, setting your limits early and resolving the situation before things get out of control may spare you significant problems and hassle. Learning how to read and understand the motivations of people will help you better identify, avoid, or deal with the *Tyrannosaurus colleagi* and, at the same time, find and appreciate the other more pleasant species of the jungle.

> **? DID YOU KNOW?**
>
> ## Help for doctors, too
>
> In many states, the state medical society has a subdivision or subsidiary that offers help to physicians with problems. The service is commonly called something like "Physician Health Services." Typically, the services were created to help physicians with alcohol and drug abuse problems. Now, however, they also offer services to physicians with behavioral problems, such as uncontrollable tempers, difficulty coping with stress, or even sexually-oriented behavior with patients and staff. The services offered are totally confidential and most state medical licensing boards are supportive of physicians enrolled in one of these programs. For more information, contact your state medical society.

Notes

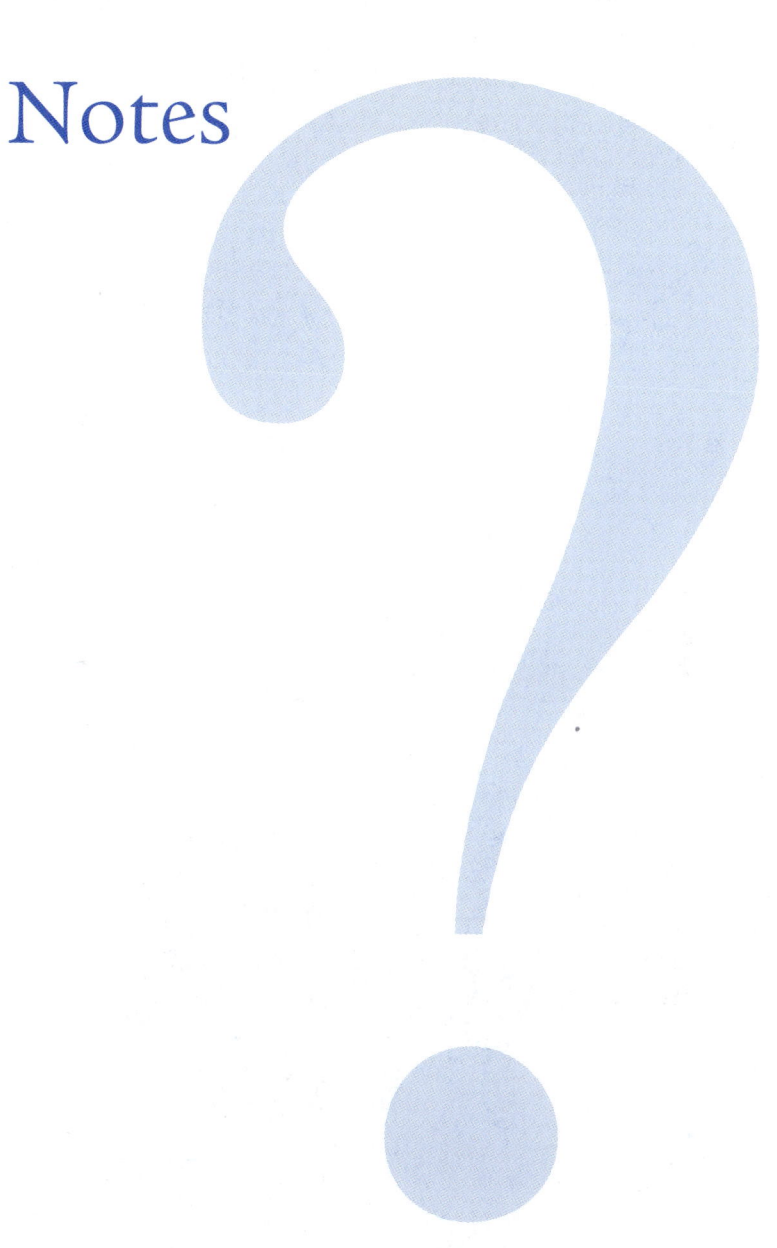

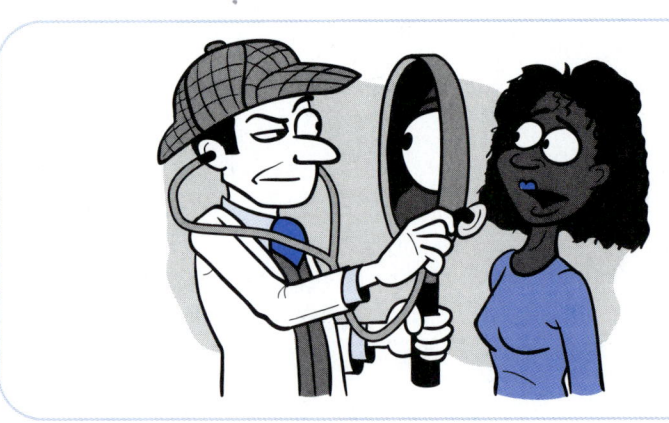

What if . . .?

It's your first day in class or your residency and you feel your acceptance was an error and you don't belong there?

In multiple interviews and discussions with medical students, residents, and practicing physicians, we've found that feeling like you don't belong is more common than you might think. You may feel there has been some mistake, a mix-up in names perhaps, and you really aren't qualified to be there. Perhaps you think your new classmates must have all attended five-star colleges and have 4.0 averages. Your puny 3.76 falls way short. How long will you last? How long before they discover the mistake and ask you to leave? That would be so embarrassing! Maybe you should just discreetly slip out the back door before they notice you.

What To Do

STOP! STOP! STOP those ridiculous thoughts immediately! Take your first lesson in how to be a health professional: the art of *trained observation*. Take a good look around you. Your new classmates are your new colleagues. Who are these people? Look closely. Is there something oddly familiar about them? No? Well, then look again *more* closely. Do you notice anyone who reminds you of a past acquaintance? How about the guy with the slicked-back hair and the shirt that is half untucked? He looks a lot like the guy in your high school class who flunked ninth grade, twice! Those three jokers in the back of the group—making noise and punching each other in the arm—are going to be doctors?! Look at the person next to you who hasn't said a word. He's biting his lip so hard it's starting to bleed! Guess what; you're probably the smartest person in the class! Besides, statistics show that even if you have the highest grades in Biochemistry and the lowest in Anatomy, the point spread from highest to lowest grades will most likely be only 5 points!

WARNING!!! Watch out for complacency. Once you get over this *What if* scenario, don't relax too much. You and your colleagues are all there with good reason and the capabilities to succeed. What will separate you from the pack are your motivation, desire, and perseverance. Once you're in, if you want success, it's yours! So, stop this nervous anxiety trip but don't go all the way to complacency. Just get to work and enjoy the greatest learning experience in your life!

DID YOU KNOW?

Be a trained observer

Sherlock Holmes, that great detective created by the ophthalmologist Sir Arthur Conan Doyle, is thought by many to be modeled after one of Doyle's mentors in medical training. Holmes was constantly using his abilities as a trained observer and a logical user of deductive reasoning to solve (diagnose) each mystery (case). Though Holmes's most famous saying to his friend and companion is "Elementary, my dear Watson!," he more often said to Dr. Watson, "Watson, you see but you do not observe!" First and foremost, a health professional must be a trained observer.

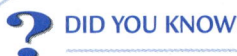

Prevention and Preparation

As you're heading into your first day in medical school, remind yourself that in order to get to this point, you had to accomplish a lot and had to excel in many ways. The competition is over. The object is to work hard and learn as much as you possibly can in order to be a good physician. Your focus should be on you and not on your colleagues.

Notes

ZZZZZ

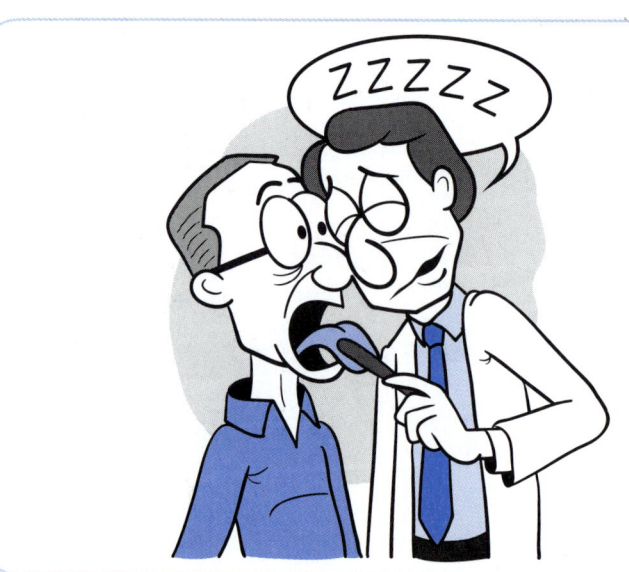

What if . . .

You have been up too many hours and are having trouble thinking?

Many of us have seen the "comical" problems sleep deprivation can cause: tired post-call interns try to unlock someone else's car in the parking lot, come out of call rooms with their clothes on backwards, fall asleep while leaning against walls, and put cream and sugar in their sodas. But sleep deprivation can have serious consequences. Various studies have shown that sleep deprivation can affect your manual dexterity, cognition, and general performance, which ultimately can harm you, your patients, and your colleagues.

Worst of all, your judgment may be impaired. Sometimes tired physicians don't even realize how they're being affected. Of course, sleepiness and weariness are signs. However, some students may argue that they're always fatigued. Watch out for decreases in attention span and initiative, lapses in memory and judgment, and increases in irritability. Be wary when you exhibit strange behaviors, such as repeating things, having to constantly re-check your work, forgetting people's names, and feeling inappropriate emotions.

Medical students are commonly afraid to reveal how tired they are, fearing that it's a sign of weakness or laziness and may negatively affect their evaluations and grades. Moreover, the culture of medicine commonly promotes staying awake, even when there is an opportunity to nap. However, most attendings and residents would rather know that the medical student is tired. They realize from personal experience what sleep deprivation can cause and would rather not deal with the consequences. In addition, the culture appears to be changing. According to a September 2002 article in *JAMA,* medical errors and motor vehicle accidents among residents have prompted restrictions on resident work hours and stimulated discussions about the importance of adequate rest and sleep.

What To Do

If possible, get sleep. Let your team know that you're having trouble thinking, and they may send you home or allow you to catch a quick nap. If circumstances don't allow you to sleep, your team can be more vigilant, provide more supervision, and assign you easier tasks to protect you, themselves, and your patients.

If your team isn't available and you have time to rest, do so—but make sure you either set an alarm or have some mechanism to prevent yourself from sleeping too long. If you don't have time to rest, let someone available know that you're struggling. It could be a nurse, a resident on another team, or another medical student that you trust. Remember you're not alone.

Also, avoid making major decisions. There are probably better times to choose where to invest all your life savings or whom to marry. Don't perform procedures that involve sharp objects and body fluids that may transmit disease or that may harm patients. Avoid driving; get a ride or take public transportation, if possible.

If you're in the middle of a procedure, stop immediately, if possible, and try to take a break. Don't continue, hoping that the "sleepiness" will pass. If you're interviewing a patient or talking to a patient's family member, politely excuse yourself. It's probably best not to let the patient and family members know that you're struggling, as they're less likely to understand. If you're in the middle of rounds or answering questions, tell the attending that you're having problems.

Prevention and Preparation

Consider natural means to help stay awake or clear your mind. Sometimes exposure to daylight, moderate exercise, or temperature change will help. A brief walk outside, jogging up and down the stairs, taking a shower, splashing cold water on your face, or drinking hot liquids are potential strategies to prevent sleep deprivation from taking over. Of course, many people rely on imbibing caffeine via coffee or soda to stay awake. However, do so cautiously because caffeine can play havoc on the normal sleep-wake cycle and the bladder.

On nights when you aren't in the hospital, make sleep a priority. When bedtime comes, drop everything you're doing and hit the sack. Make sure your bedroom is quiet, dark, and cool (temperature-wise) enough to sleep. Avoid stimulants, such as caffeine, large meals, and annoying people, right before bedtime. Having a daily relaxing ritual (such as reading this book or meditating) before bedtime can help.

In general, treat sleep deprivation as you would intoxication or impairment. Take the necessary precautions and try to treat the impairment as soon as possible. If you don't realize the importance of sleep, it's best to sleep on this *What if* until you do!

What if . . .

You're failing or failed a course in medical school?

Failure is a part of life. Anyone who claims to have never failed is failing to tell the truth or failing to leave the house. Many successful entrepreneurs, scientists, actors, and artists floundered before hitting the jackpot. The list of highly successful people who suffered significant career mishaps is long and includes Michael Jordan, Albert Einstein, Donald Trump, and Ashley Judd.

Unfortunately, super-achieving medical students and physicians commonly have expectations of themselves and others that are far too high. In some cases, these expectations can contribute to an environment of excellence; in others, though, they can be detrimental. Failure in itself isn't bad. On the contrary, it can be instructive, build character, and even save lives—but only if you understand the causes of that failure and potential solutions. Moreover, failing one course won't sink your career. Reasonable people understand that missteps happen and look for trends instead of isolated incidents. (Would you start a blood pressure medication for a single high reading?)

What To Do

Be a problem solver. Be honest with yourself in determining why you might have failed or are failing; the answers you come up with may point you toward a solution. Remember, you can't change the past but you can learn from it. Focus your actions on how to recognize and fix the problem if it happens again.

The Human Evaluator

Not surprisingly, course evaluation is commonly subjective, especially during your third year of medical school. Random impressions, personal bias, and bad luck can influence the evaluator. Even the most fabulous medical student may stutter through a presentation, spill coffee on the attending's jacket, or be paralyzed by anxiety. If you aren't able to put your best foot forward, consider discussing these issues with your evaluator. Certainly double-check to make sure no obvious grading errors have occurred. Your evaluators are human (believe it or not) and do make mistakes.

However, be fair to your evaluator. If no obvious errors have occurred, don't claim errors occurred or dwell on the possibility. Also, don't complain about the grading system or the teaching after the grade has been issued when it's too late to change these factors. Too many students stay clear of the evaluators throughout the course but then line up to see them after the course ends when their grades aren't what they expected.

Good, Bad, and Ugly

Alternatively, your concentration could have been affected by external circumstances, ranging from such minor distractions as friends and video games to more serious crises, such as a death in the family and relationship difficulties. Academic difficulties may be early indicators of persistent personal problems. Determine how major and correctable these circumstances are. Focus on resolving the situation. As in clinical medicine, simply treating the symptoms won't solve the underlying problem. If the problem is major, don't try to be superhuman and conduct business as usual. Get help if needed. Consider explaining your situation to the course director. Although, in general, you should be conscientious about your coursework, there are more important aspects of life that shouldn't be ignored.

 WARNING!!! Don't wallow in your defeat. Everyone is entitled to a short period of shock, anger, or disappointment but don't let it hamper you from solving the problem that led to your failure. Don't automatically blame the test, grading system, or evaluators. Yes, they can all be unfair. However, unless they're biased specifically against you and can be changed, it isn't productive to blame them. Of course, there are situations where obvious inequities occurred. If an oral examiner or evaluator has a history of disliking you and treating you unfairly, you may request another examiner. If your copy of the test didn't have the correct instructions or you weren't given the same amount of time as other students to complete the exam, then you may request a re-test. If other students received credit for answers that you provided but didn't receive credit for, you may request a re-grade.

Prevention and Preparation

In addition to addressing problems when you're failing a course, here are some ways to prevent getting into a near-failing situation.

The Right Stuff

Sometimes success is about more than knowing the facts. Maybe you didn't study the right material, adequately prepare, or tailor your preparation to the type of exam. (For example, if the exam involves solving patient cases, simply memorizing facts may not be enough.) Knowing the material doesn't guarantee doing well in a class. Seek advice from other students, faculty, or the course director about what material to focus on and how to best prepare. Also, find out how you're being evaluated.

Nose to the Grindstone

Perhaps the skills required by the course aren't your strong suit. Maybe, for you, studying microbiology is like Tiger Woods playing a linebacker. Instead of railing against your disadvantage, simply accept that you may have to work harder than others to compensate.

A Frame-Up

Apathy can also lead to poor performance. For example, a future radiologist may not see the immediate relevance of a psychiatry course. In such cases, try to mentally frame the course in a way that is interesting and relevant to you. For example, psychiatrists order brain imaging studies, which are carried out by radiologists. What's more, psychiatry is involved in all human interactions with colleagues, friends, and in-laws—especially in-laws.

Stay in the Game

Remember medical education and training is a marathon, not a sprint. If you fall, there is plenty of time to get up and finish the race. Just make sure you figure out why you fell and how to avoid it down the road, wear good shoes, and drink plenty of fluids and you can handle this *What if* scenario like a pro.

What if . . . ?

Emergency!

What if . . .

You're starting an IV and the catheter breaks off in the vein?

Aside from a few well-packaged items in the cafeteria and some of the duller-edged greeting cards in the gift shop, nothing is completely safe in the hospital. Even starting an intravenous (IV) line, which is done dozens or even hundreds of times each day in any medical center, can have its dangers. Intravenous catheter placement can result in infection, cause or dislodge blood clots, and puncture arteries. Moreover, pieces of the catheter can break off and travel through the vein into the heart and pulmonary circulation. There, it can lodge itself in the heart, causing abnormal heart rhythms or heart attacks or block the circulation of blood to parts of the lung, potentially leading to serious problems and even death.

Therefore, even though you consider yourself a well-seasoned veteran at IV line placement, be careful and vigilant each time you do it. It only takes one mistake, one defective catheter, or one unfortunate event for the catheter to break.

What To Do

If you encounter resistance when removing an IV line, stop pulling, cover the area with sterile bandages or pads to prevent infection, and apply warm compresses to the area to relax the vein. After a short while, try removing the line again. If you still have resistance, contact vascular surgery or interventional radiology immediately.

If the catheter breaks, your goal is to prevent the broken piece from migrating up the vein to the patient's pulmonary circulation and heart. Keep the arm still and below the level of the heart. Place a venous tourniquet around the patient's arm close to his or her armpit (axillary area) to inhibit the piece from flowing through the vein toward the heart. Check the patient's wrist pulse to ensure that the tourniquet isn't so tight that it blocks blood flow to the patient's arm. Don't inject anything into the broken catheter. Immediately contact vascular surgery or interventional radiology to remove the piece. Don't attempt to remove it yourself.

 WARNING!!! Leakage of fluid or a popping, burning, or stinging sensation in the patient's arm when fluid passes through the IV line suggests that the catheter is torn.

Prevention and Preparation

To avoid this mishap, use catheters carefully and properly. Don't cut, twist, or overmanipulate them. When injecting fluid into the catheter, don't apply too much pressure. Because the size of the injection syringe barrel is inversely proportional to the amount of pressure applied to the catheter (smaller barrel, greater pressure), you should refrain from using syringes that are too small for the catheter you're using. (For example, for a PICC line, you shouldn't use a syringe smaller than 10 mL.)

Carefully inspect the catheter for breaks and damage before using it. Keep scissors and other sharp objects away from the catheter.

Of course, hundreds of IV lines are started each day without complications. You shouldn't be paranoid; just don't take seemingly simple procedures for granted. Take a cue from Tiger Woods, who takes every short putt seriously, and Michael Jordan, who tried to concentrate on every single free throw, and remember that there is no such thing as a "gimme" or a "no-brainer."

What if . . .

You get stuck with a dirty needle?

It isn't uncommon for a health-care worker to get stuck accidentally by a dirty needle or be exposed to a patient's body secretions. Of the diseases that may be contracted, HIV, hepatitis B virus (HBV), and hepatitis C virus (HCV) are among the most serious. Even so, the transmission rates for HIV are low: less than 0.3% from a percutaneous exposure and less than 0.1% for a mucocutaneous exposure. The use of postexposure prophylaxis (PEP) has reduced HIV transmission by about 80%. The transmission rate for HBV after a needlestick is much higher: 6% to 30% in those health-care workers not immune to HBV, although preexposure vaccination or prior infection eliminates the risk of transmission. The incidence of HCV transmission is approximately 1.8% per injury with a range of 0% to 7%.

What To Do

Early initiation of PEP is critical for it to work, so you should seek treatment immediately at your occupational health office or the Emergency Department after an exposure. The Centers for Disease Control and Prevention provides specific guidelines for PEP for HIV and recommends that PEP be administered to health-care workers exposed to HIV under certain circumstances. A complete listing of these guidelines can be found at *http://www.cdc.gov/mmwr/preview/mmwrhtml/rr5011a1.htm*.

The decision to use PEP hinges on an assessment of the exposure risk and the HIV status of the source patient. Exposures that are considered to have a higher risk of transmission include exposure to a larger amount of blood, a visibly bloody device, injury with a needle used in a patient's vein or artery, and a deep injury. Source patients who are considered a high risk include patients with late-stage HIV and those with high HIV titers and increased viral load.

 WARNING!!! Although the previous guidelines give a general idea of how to gauge when PEP is appropriate, remember that the decision to administer PEP should be made on a case-by-case basis.

Combination therapy with zidovudine and lamivudine is currently recommended for most PEP for HIV. A three-drug regimen (adding stavudine or didanosine to the two-drug combination) is recommended for exposures with the highest risk. Guidelines suggest starting PEP as soon as possible—within 1 to 2 hours—and usually restrict therapy to within 36 hours of exposure, although therapy may be given more than 36 hours after exposure in high-risk situations.

Health-care workers who aren't immune to HBV may be treated with hepatitis B immune globulin and the hepatitis B vaccine should be initiated. This combination is more than 90% effective in preventing HBV. At this point, there is no vaccine available to prevent HCV and no recommended treatment with PEP. Those health-care workers with known exposure to HCV should be monitored for seroconversion.

Prevention and Preparation

Many patients may have unsuspected HIV or hepatitis infection, so you should follow standard precautions at all times. You can significantly decrease your risk of exposure to infectious pathogens by using protective equipment, such as gloves, a gown, eye protection, and a facemask in any situation where an exposure may occur. To decrease needlesticks, use devices with safety features if available, avoid recapping needles, and dispose of used needles promptly in appropriate containers. As a health-care worker, you should be immunized with the hepatitis B vaccine to prevent this disease. If you suspect that you've been exposed or if you have questions about possible exposure to HIV, HBV, HCV or other diseases, call the National Clinicians' Post-Exposure Prophylaxis Hotline at 1-888-HIV-4911.

Notes

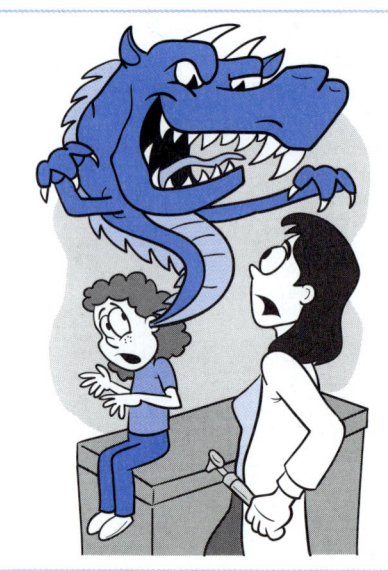

What if . . .

A patient has a cockroach or similar insect in her ear canal?

People—especially children—stick lots of strange things in their ears, ranging from beads and toys to vegetable matter. Insects can also unexpectedly crawl into the ear while people are sleeping. When an insect is involved, a patient usually feels the insect moving, hears a buzzing sound, or just feels something in the ear. The cockroach is the most common ear-nesting culprit in the United States. Complications of an insect or other foreign body in the ear canal include ear canal lacerations (usually from attempts to remove the insect), otitis externa, and tympanic membrane perforation.

What To Do

First, you must ask the patient if she tried to remove the insect. Such an attempt may have injured the ear canal or perforated the tympanic membrane. If the tympanic membrane is perforated, you should not be using any of the irrigation techniques or insect-anesthetizing techniques that follow. To check for injury or perforation, straighten the canal by grasping the pinna of the ear and gently pulling it up and back. A speculum of adequate size and a sufficient light source are necessary for an adequate view. You should visualize the tympanic membrane to make sure it isn't perforated before you attempt to remove the insect.

To prevent or minimize patient anxiety, explain what you have found in a very reassuring manner. Because an insect in the ear canal may produce physical discomfort as well as marked anxiety, the patient—especially a child—may require sedation to some degree. For a young child, conscious sedation or even general anesthesia may be necessary to make her comfortable, minimize trauma during removal, and avoid pushing the insect further into the canal.

To allow for easier removal, the insect should first be immobilized. Various agents can be used, including 2% lidocaine or mineral oil with lidocaine and alcohol.

WARNING!!! Do not use these agents if the tympanic membrane is perforated. You will need the help of an otolaryngologist.

Removing the insect from the ear canal may be accomplished using various methods:

- *Forceps.* Use forceps, such as alligator forceps, to grasp the insect and pull it out.
- *Blunt hook.* Under direct visualization, pass a blunt hook behind the insect to ease it out of the canal.
- *Suction.* Use suction with a small catheter to suck the insect out of the canal.
- *Irrigation.* Unless the tympanic membrane is perforated or you suspect it might be, use room temperature or warm water and an IV catheter to irrigate the canal.

WARNING!!! Using cold water will cause severe nausea or even vomiting. Aim the irrigation fluid at the periphery of the insect in order to hit the tympanic membrane and create a backpressure to push the in-

WATCH OUT FOR...

Potentially hysterical patient

Many people are extremely fearful of insects and could easily become hysterical upon being informed that there is a cockroach in their ear. It becomes very difficult to say, "Please hold still while I remove it." Instead of alarming the patient, say something like, "It appears there is a foreign body lodged in the ear canal. It should be a simple matter for me to remove it and clear the canal." After you have successfully removed the "foreign body," you can then explain to them what it was.

In reality, it's hard to be certain about what the foreign body is until you have removed it and can closely inspect it. So prematurely informing the patient may not only alarm them, but could also be providing misinformation and alarming them unnecessarily.

sect out of the canal. (In addition to membrane perforation, avoid irrigation of foreign bodies that may swell when wet, such as plant material.)

After removing the insect, examine the ear canal again for any damage or retained material. If you can't remove an impacted foreign body in the ear canal, you should seek assistance from an otolaryngologist.

Prevention and Preparation

Unfortunately, prevention of insects entering the ear canal is difficult as they usually enter the canal when you're sleeping. A good exterminator may be the best prevention. If the patient's living circumstances are such that it's unlikely the insect infestation can be eliminated from the environment, you may want to suggest that the patient sleep with soft ear plugs in place. Finally, when you start to evaluate a patient complaining of ear symptoms, remember this *What if* and be prepared for anything smaller than your elbow!

What if . . .

A patient, friend, or family member has a tick burrowed into his skin?

Tick bites most commonly occur in the spring and summer and are responsible for many different diseases that vary by geographic region. Tick-borne diseases include Lyme disease, Rocky Mountain spotted fever, ehrlichiosis, tularemia, babesiosis, relapsing fever, and Colorado tick fever. These diseases should be considered if a patient has a nonspecific febrile illness, especially with a rash present that occurs after a tick bite. However, many people don't realize they've been bitten by a tick. Most of the ticks that transmit disease are so-called "deer ticks," which are very tiny and difficult to see unless their bodies are engorged with the patient's blood. So don't rule out a tick-borne illness if your patient doesn't recall being bitten by a tick. If your patient has a rash or rash and a fever, inspect the usual locations (arms, legs, and torso, especially around the belt-line), for signs of an insect bite.

What To Do

To remove a tick embedded in a person's skin, first apply viscous lidocaine to kill the tick and numb the area. Then use forceps to apply gentle traction to the tick's head and carefully remove the tick. Be careful to remove all parts of the tick as leaving residual body parts can lead to infection. After removing the tick, thoroughly disinfect the bite site and wash your hands with soap and water.

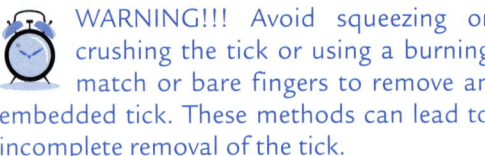 WARNING!!! Avoid squeezing or crushing the tick or using a burning match or bare fingers to remove an embedded tick. These methods can lead to incomplete removal of the tick.

If you or a friend has sustained a tick bite and goes on to develop fever or rash, you should seek medical care to be evaluated for a tick-borne disease. Antibiotics can successfully treat many tick-borne diseases.

Prevention and Preparation

If you can't avoid a tick-infested area, use skin and clothing repellents to avoid being bitten. Permethrin is a pesticide that may be used as a clothing spray to protect against ticks. The best way to avoid a tick bite is by wearing protective clothing treated with permethrin in combination with using a topical insect repellent on exposed skin. After outdoor exposure, be sure to check yourself for ticks.

WATCH OUT FOR...
Rash without a tick

Rashes without an obvious tick may still be due to tick-borne disease. In obtaining the history of the present illness, ask about exposure in settings where ticks are common: rolling in the grass, long walks through brush, exposure to pets infested with ticks, or recently spending time in an endemic area (such as the south coast of New England, Martha's Vineyard, Nantucket Island, and many more).

In the early stages of Lyme disease, the initial lesion may look like a spider bite, especially if the tick has disengaged and departed. When treating a lesion as a probable spider bite, follow up with the patient 4 to 7 days later. You may see the central papule has disappeared and the advancing arc of erythema migrans, the classic Lyme disease rash, is quite obvious.

Notes

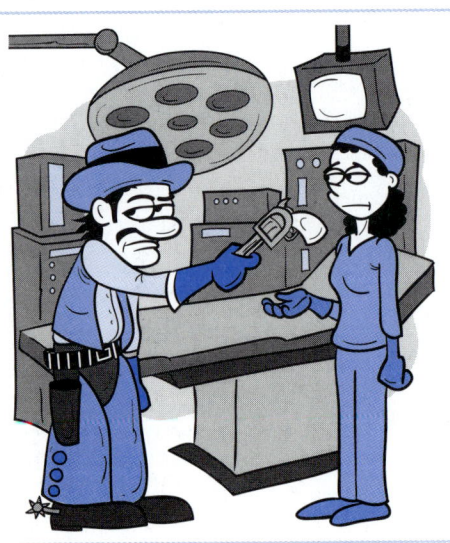

What if . . .

You're examining a patient in the Emergency Department and you discover a gun tucked in his waistband (belt)?

With the prevalence of street gangs these days, it wouldn't be that unusual to be faced with this *What if* scenario. The patient may be the victim of violence or may just be suffering from a medical illness. Much more commonly, the patient is a law enforcement officer and licensed to carry such a weapon. Regardless, you must take specific steps.

What To Do

Don't panic. The simplest thing to do is to say calmly, "I notice you have a weapon. Why would that be? I'm uncomfortable examining and treating you with the weapon present. Would you be willing to temporarily surrender it to our security staff?"

If the patient is accompanied by a friend or family member, he might be willing to have that person take the gun away. If the patient agrees to surrender his weapon (and most will), step out of the room to call the security officer for your facility. Of course, you should explain to the patient that you're calling security. Even if the patient is a law enforcement officer, have him surrender the weapon to security. When the weapon has been surrendered and secured, you can proceed with examining and treating the patient.

If the patient is unconscious, contact your facility's security department and request assistance. It's best to have someone who's licensed to carry a weapon remove it from an unconscious patient. Most health-care facilities require their security personnel to be licensed to carry a weapon, even if they don't carry a weapon while on duty.

When it's time to return the weapon to the patient, the security staff should do that. It's usually standard policy and practice for the security staff to then ask the patient if they have a license to carry the weapon, before they give the weapon back to the patient. If the patient doesn't have a license, the security officer won't return the weapon to the patient, but will instead surrender it to the local police.

If the patient refuses to surrender the weapon, simply state, "I'm really sorry, but I'm uncomfortable and won't be able to treat you today." Politely ask the patient to leave and excuse yourself from the examination room.

Alternative Action

If you're uncomfortable speaking with the patient about the weapon, simply state, "I notice you're carrying a weapon. I'm required to ask our security people to speak with you about it. Excuse me while I notify them." Then calmly exit to call security.

Prevention and Preparation

Because the most common scenario involves the patient who's a law enforcement officer, it can be helpful if your facility periodically communicates a "No weapons policy" to local law enforcement agencies. You should also familiarize yourself with your facility's policy and procedure for addressing this situation. Finally, always commit to memory the number to call for security for the facility in which you're working.

What if . . . You're resuscitating a patient in a hospital and there is a gunman loose in the hallways?

This scenario could easily happen, particularly if the patient you're resuscitating is a victim of violence. If the crime is gang-related, the perpetrator may have entered the hospital to finish the job of killing the victim. Now, you may be thinking, "If I were resuscitating a patient, how would I know there was a gunman loose in the hallways?" One possible way would be having it reported to you during the resuscitation. If the patient is the victim of violence, another source of information may be the patient's friend or family member who accompanied them into the treatment room. The friend or family member may tell you that the perpetrator is likely to come into the hospital to "finish the job."

What To Do

If the information about the gunman is reported to you from outside the treatment room, it implies that key people in the hospital are aware of the situation and the danger. You're actions, in addition to continuing to be in charge of the resuscitation of the patient, are to issue orders to secure and lock the room you're working in (if possible) and to secure and lock-down the Emergency Department. Ask someone to make sure that the security department is aware of the situation. Ask someone to get a security guard posted outside the room you're in. Don't stop the resuscitation while doing so. Issue such orders, as the person in charge of the resuscitation. Realize that this situation is no different from issuing orders for IV fluids or medications during resuscitation.

If the information about a gunman or potential gunman comes from the patient's friend or family member, you must act to notify someone. Again, issue orders as the person in charge. Ask someone immediately to call the security department to inform them of the situation. Request that the room you're in be locked (if possible), that the Emergency Department be secured and locked down, and that the waiting area be cleared. The patient's immediate family or accompanying friend should be sequestered in a safe area. The security personnel will call the local police in such a situation. Continue resuscitating the patient. With these efforts, it's unlikely that a gunman will get to your area. If the gunman gains access to your treatment area, there isn't much you can do except cooperate with him. Cooperation may mean discontinuing the resuscitation and losing a life, but that action may save several other lives including your own.

It's important to realize that most hospital security department personnel are unarmed and fairly defenseless against an armed perpetrator. So security usually acts quickly to summon local police in such a scenario. However, on the plus side, hospitals that do have armed security guards are usually the hospitals with the greatest potential for dangerous crime occurring in the hospital. Keep in mind, a security guard isn't likely to take a bullet to save a "John Doe," and neither should you.

Prevention and Preparation

There is little you can do to prevent this scenario from occurring, but there are some things you can do to be better prepared. If you're working in an emergency department or frequently get called to go to the emergency department, familiarize yourself with security procedures and policy. Ask those in charge how such situations are usually handled. Speak with the security guards to get advice from them about the best actions to take. If the people you're speaking with express surprise or uncertainty (which is unlikely), take the time to explain your concerns and your desire to know and understand security procedures for the emergency department. Make sure that they understand you want to be of assistance, not a critic and not an additional problem for them to deal with during a crisis.

What if . . . Your morbidly obese patient needs a venous cutdown or other invasive procedure?

Obesity not only raises the risk of having many diseases, including heart disease and diabetes, but also makes it more difficult to perform medical procedures. Morbidly obese patients are commonly too large and heavy to fit in or on conventional medical equipment, such as stretchers, exam tables, and imaging machines. Large amounts of fat can make it difficult to find and access certain parts of the body. Physicians rely on seeing and feeling different body structures to guide where they place needles, scalpels, catheters, and tubes. There is typically only a very small margin for error. Miss the body structure, and you may obtain the wrong tissue or body fluid, deliver medication to the wrong location, or puncture a vital structure.

What To Do

If you can't see the clear anatomic landmarks to perform a procedure, use available imaging devices to help guide you. It's too risky to go "fishing" for the vein, artery, or whatever you're trying to reach. An ultrasound machine can usually show adequate anatomic detail. If you aren't experienced in using an ultrasound machine, find someone who is. Ultrasound pictures can be very confusing when you first see them, looking like television screen fuzz. Someone else can move the ultrasound probe, interpret the pictures, and guide you while you perform the procedure.

Live and In Person

Ultrasound isn't good, however, at showing areas that have a lot of air (such as the lungs and intestines) or bone (below the outer surfaces of the bone). Sometimes even ultrasound can't penetrate large amounts of body tissue. Therefore, fluoroscopy, or "live" x-ray imaging, may be needed to find your target. In fluoroscopy, pressing a switch turns on an x-ray beam that is transmitted through the patient to create a real-time, moving x-ray image on a television screen. Fluoroscopy can be performed only by those properly certified in the procedure. Therefore, you'll have to ask a radiologist, cardiologist, surgeon, or other appropriate specialist (depending on the procedure) to perform the imaging and procedure. When fluoroscopy can't provide enough guidance, computed tomography (CT) or magnetic resonance imaging (MRI) can show certain muscles, organs, and soft tissue more clearly and may help guide procedures. When all of this fails, surgeons may have to take the patient to the operating room to perform the procedure under general anesthesia.

 WARNING!!! While the patient's size may make procedures difficult and inconvenient, be careful not to show frustration or any expressions that may offend the patient. The patient certainly doesn't intend to create hassles.

Prevention and Preparation

Anticipate what procedures may need to be done for the patient and schedule them with

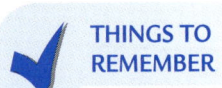 **THINGS TO REMEMBER**

Radiology strategies

Whenever a morbidly obese patient needs radiological imaging, make sure you inform the radiologists or radiology department about the patient's size and weight. They may need to use several strategies, including:

- using special imaging exam tables that can hold heavier patients.
- using extra-large imaging equipment as some patients are too large to fit inside traditional computed tomography and magnetic resonance imaging machines.
- using special transportation devices that are sturdy and large enough to bring the patient to the imaging room.
- increasing electrical current or radiation exposure to penetrate the body tissue.

the appropriate specialists as soon as possible. When you contact the specialist, make sure you clearly describe the patient's location and body size as well as the nature and urgency of the procedure. Procedures can be delayed if the scheduler doesn't realize the urgency of the procedure or the wrong kind of imaging equipment is used. Sometimes imaging equipment specially designed to handle larger patients will be needed. If you anticipate that the patient will require several procedures, try to get them accomplished all at the same time, while the imaging equipment or specialists are available. As you can see, treating morbidly obese patients can require significant planning and coordination. As the rate of obesity in the general population continues to rise, this problem will become more common—and preparing for this *What if* will be a good investment of your time!

What if . . .

Someone collapses at a social function you're attending?

Odds are, this *What if* will definitely happen to you if it hasn't already. The person, or *victim* as they're usually referred to, may lose consciousness completely due to a syncopal episode caused by a vasovagal reaction (see the *What if* on page 119), cardiac arrhythmia or, perhaps, a central nervous system (CNS) event, such as a stroke or seizure. Alternatively, the victim may simply sink to the floor but remain conscious, though confused or poorly responsive. Regardless of the cause or exact condition, as a physician or physician-in-training, or other health professional, people who know you will expect you to know what to do.

What To Do

You must first assess the situation, gather information, and draw preliminary conclusions. Then take specific action. Unfortunately, most people will expect you to skip directly to the action. Buy some time to evaluate the victim and relieve pressure to take immediate action by approaching the victim promptly, getting him or her fully recumbent, elevating the head very slightly, and taking the victim's pulse. You need this information anyway and it looks to observers as if you're taking action.

While taking the pulse, start observing as much as you can. Use your eyes and nose to gather information. Is the victim breathing? Is the skin pale and clammy or reddened and flushed? Is there a health-warning bracelet on the victim's wrist? People with diabetes or seizure disorders commonly wear medical identification jewelry to aid first responders if such an event occurs. Is there any sign of injury? Check the pupils. Speak to the victim to solicit a response. Identify yourself as a health professional and tell him or her what you're doing to help. What odors do you detect? Alcohol? Ketones?

Establishing the presence or absence of a pulse is crucial. No pulse means you must begin cardiopulmonary resuscitation (CPR) and send someone to call 911. If you're in a public facility, such as an airport, theatre, or shopping mall, ask specifically for someone to call 911 and also for an automatic external defibrillator (AED). Increasingly, public facilities are equipped with one or more AEDs (see *What if* on page 129).

If the victim has a pulse, determine the rate and note any irregularity in the rhythm. Determine the heart rate. (Rates below 40 or above 200 may cause significant hypotension.) If the patient has a pulse and is unconscious and motionless, it's likely the result of a syncopal episode due to a transitory hypotensive period. The recumbent position should enable the victim to gradually regain consciousness. If the patient doesn't regain consciousness and the heart rate is normal, something is probably affecting the CNS, such as a stroke, cerebral hemorrhage, drug or alcohol intoxication, severe hypoglycemia, or even a seizure disorder. If seizurelike activity is present (tonic-clonic muscle contractions), position the victim on his or her side and protect him or her from injury.

 WARNING!!! Don't try to insert anything into a seizing person's mouth. Doing so risks injury to the victim and, possibly, yourself or others.

 **DID YOU KNOW?**

The difference AEDs can make

Approximately 1000 deaths occur daily in the United States due to cardiac arrest outside the hospital setting. Most of these cardiac arrests are a result of ventricular fibrillation, which is usually fatal within minutes. Studies show that the probability of survival from cardiac arrest outside the hospital is about 5% if normal sinus rhythm isn't achieved within 10 minutes. Immediately available AEDs can make a difference.

Prevention and Preparation

Think about this scenario in advance. It will happen to you eventually. Take an appropriate course and become certified in Basic Life Support (CPR). Familiarize yourself with one of the typical AEDs. When you're in that public setting, waiting for the game to start, waiting for the plane to arrive, or waiting in a line, imagine the scenario develops and what your first actions would be.

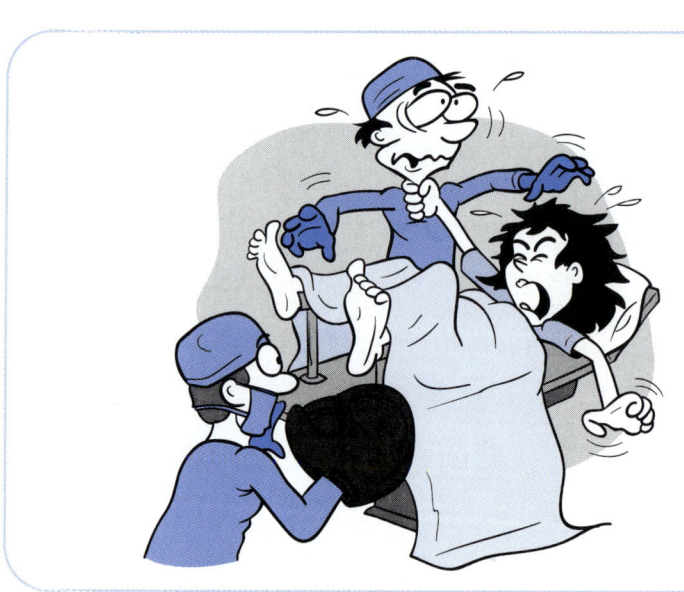

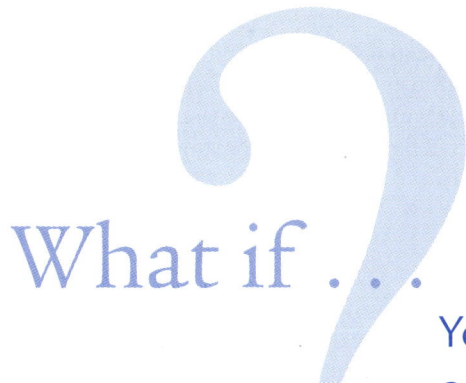

What if . . .

You have to deliver a baby outside the hospital?

There are three stages of labor and delivery:

- *Stage 1* involves cervical dilation and effacement with uterine contractions and is usually the longest—up to 12 hours. Active labor occurs when contractions become regular and rhythmic, occur at least 5 minutes apart, and last for at least 60 seconds.
- *Stage 2* is the actual delivery of the baby and begins with the baby's head stretching the vagina and the perineum, causing the mother's urge to push or bear down. She shouldn't start pushing until the widest part of the baby's head appears at the vaginal opening (called *crowning*) because pushing before crowning will cause the partially dilated cervix to become edematous.
- *Stage 3* occurs after the baby is born. During this stage, the uterus contracts again to deliver the placenta. Bleeding during this time may persist, but shouldn't be excessive.

Next Stop, Outside the Textbook

Although the previous scenario is typical, the birth of a baby can't be predicted to such a degree. As you've seen in movies and on television, birth can happen anywhere, such as in a taxicab, at home, and at the supermarket. Such a situation will be drastically different from the sterile medical environment you might be familiar with: the mother lying in a hospital bed with her legs in stirrups surrounded by a physician or midwife and nurses. In any case, you may easily find yourself present at such an unpredicted birth where your medical expertise will almost certainly be needed.

What To Do

Mom is anxious enough for everyone involved; so, obviously, you must be the calm one. Let mom know that you have medical training and are familiar with delivering babies. Most importantly, do NOT boil water, which is a common myth about childbirth that was most likely constructed to keep uninitiated fathers out from underfoot. Instead, calmly instruct the mother to breathe deeply (but not to push!) and call 911 from the nearest phone. When you call, try to have answers to these questions:

- When did the amniotic sac rupture (the water break)?
- Was there a foul odor or greenish-black color to the amniotic fluid? (Distressed babies may stain the amniotic fluid with stool, or *meconium*.)
- How far apart are the contractions and how long do they last?
- Is there associated bloody discharge?

While waiting for paramedics, make sure that the mom is lying comfortably and safely on a flat, cushioned surface—such as the backseat of a car, a blanket on the floor, or a bed or sofa. Next, grab several pillows or roll several blankets to prop against mom's right side, so that she's leaning slightly to her left side, which physically lifts the baby off mom's abdominal vena cava and improves her circulation. Instruct her to resist the urge to push, which can be very difficult and painful (like resisting the pressure of an impending bowel movement!),

THINGS TO REMEMBER

When you deliver a baby

- Keep the mother and baby warm and dry.
- The umbilical cord may strangulate the baby during delivery by blocking its blood and oxygen supply, so it *must* be unraveled from the neck as early as possible.
- Cutting the umbilical cord or injuring the placenta may cause significant bleeding in both patients. Leave these procedures for the doctors at the hospital.
- Stimulation from breastfeeding will help control the vaginal bleeding caused by the delivery.

and to take regular, deep breaths. Also—and this is NOT a myth—have plenty of towels and blankets readily available because childbirth is a messy process. Towels can keep mom and the newborn warm and wipe away all sorts of substances that come out, such as blood, amniotic fluid, urine, and stool. Finally, you'll need to take a peek, so position the mother with her legs bent at the knees and spread open, to give you a direct view of the vagina.

They Said It's Your Birthday . . .

If, on initial examination, the baby's hair is visible (crowning), delivery is imminent. Place your palms against the head to slow delivery. Have the mom take a deep breath and push down steadily, as if making a bowel movement, for 10 seconds (counting out loud for mom can be helpful). Then have her take another breath and repeat the process. When the head is delivered, feel around the baby's neck for the umbilical cord. If the cord is wrapped around the neck, gently slip it off. If no cord is felt, with your palms cradling the baby's head and covering its ears, firmly but gently guide the baby's body from the mom with each push only. The anterior shoulder is usually delivered first, followed by the posterior shoulder.

 WARNING!!! Don't attempt to yank the baby out when the mother isn't pushing. Think of it as *catching* the baby. The mother does the *delivering* part.

Hold on Tight

After delivery, you should be holding a wet, warm, slippery bundle of arms and legs—so hold on! Promptly wipe off all the fluid and completely swathe the newborn in a warm blanket or towel. The baby should almost immediately start crying, which means that you did everything right. Leave the umbilical cord intact; cutting the cord may cause the mother and baby to bleed. Don't worry if the baby looks a little blue; it's common before they take their first breath to cry. Immediately place the baby next to the mother's skin for additional warmth and have the mother begin breastfeeding. Breast stimulation will help control the amount of vaginal bleeding caused by the delivery.

Mom may continue to experience cramping after the delivery because the placenta is still attached. The placenta is a group of blood vessels attached to the uterus that provides nutrients and oxygen to the fetus. When the placenta is delivered, place it next to the baby. Doing so may seem a little disconcerting, but the doctors at the hospital will want to examine the placenta to make sure that it's intact and nothing is left inside the uterus. Make

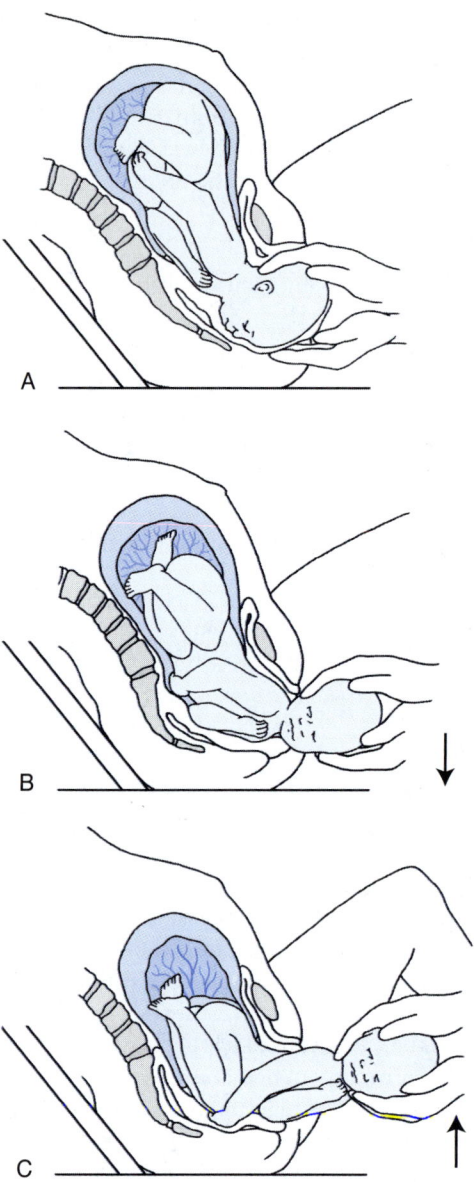

Stages of delivery. *(A)* Delivering the head. *(B)* Delivering the anterior shoulder.
(C) Delivering the posterior shoulder.

certain that mother and baby are covered and brought immediately to the hospital.

Prevention and Preparation

Avoid "termophobia" (the fear of any woman near term in a pregnancy) and the urge to leave the vicinity when it hits. Get familiar with delivering a baby. Take an OB rotation if you're still in training. Otherwise, read about the procedure, discuss it with OB-GYNs you know, and seek an opportunity to assist with some deliveries.

What if . . .

The baby you just delivered outside the hospital isn't breathing?

You think *you've* had a tough day? Chances are, the day of a newborn delivered outside a prepared birthing environment will be tougher. He starts the day in the womb with his lungs full of amniotic fluid, not having to worry about warmth or breathing. Then he travels down the birth canal, squeezing much of the amniotic fluid out of his lungs, emerges without anyone suctioning the fluid out of his nose or mouth, and copes with a suddenly colder environment. To top it off, your face is the first thing that newborn sees (which, depending on the last time you showered, may be the biggest shock). After all that, he has to breathe? That's *pressure!*

Even with such pressure, the newborn is typically stimulated to breathe by the temperature change, light, lack of oxygen without the placenta, and elastic recoil of the chest after leaving the vaginal canal. However, sometimes this stimulation isn't enough, especially for premature babies with immature lungs and small bodies easily susceptible to hypothermia.

Other conditions can inhibit that first breath. Thick meconium (the newborn's first stool) can plug his airway. Sedatives taken by his mom can suppress breathing. Bleeding from trauma or placental problems and anatomic abnormalities, such as incompletely formed airways or lungs, masses obstructing the airways, and diaphragmatic hernias, also can be culprits.

What To Do

Remain calm. Don't unnecessarily alarm the mother. Promptly dry and wrap the baby in a blanket or similar garment to prevent hypothermia. Then, position him so that he can breathe easily. Since tilting his head forward or too far backward might close off his trachea, keep his head tilted slightly backward (with the neck slightly extended) by putting a rolled diaper or small towel under his shoulders. A newborn with a meningomyelocele (exposed spinal cord or meninges due to incomplete vertebral column closure) should be placed on his side or tummy rather than his back.

Carefully remove the secretions (by positioning him on his side to let the secretions drain out of his posterior pharynx or using a clean finger or tissue) or suction them (with a suction bulb) as well as meconium, if present, from the newborn's mouth and then his nose. (Do the mouth first to prevent him from aspirating.) Suctioning too aggressively may injure him or stimulate his vagus nerve, which slows down his heart.

If he doesn't start breathing, *gently* stimulate him by flicking the bottom of his feet and rubbing his back.

Ventilate or Resuscitate

If these steps are unsuccessful, ventilate (preferably with a Bag-Valve-Mask) and transport him to the nearest emergency facility immediately. If a Bag-Valve-Mask isn't available, resuscitate using the mouth to mouth-and-nose method:

- Open his airway by gently lifting his chin.
- Inhale deeply and seal your mouth over his mouth and nose. (If you can't create a seal around his nose and mouth, try blowing into either the nose or the mouth while covering the other.)
- Blow slowly into his mouth and nose simultaneously for 1 to $1^1/_2$ seconds.
- Make sure his chest rises when you blow and falls after the breath is done.
- After you finish blowing, release your mouth, and repeat the steps (from positioning, to blowing, to releasing) at a rate of about 30 breaths per minute.

No rise in the chest

If the newborn's chest doesn't move up and down during ventilation, there may be one of several problems:

- His airway may be blocked by his:
  1. *head position.* Tilt his head slightly further backward or forward. Make sure you're lifting his chin.
  2. *secretions.* Try to re-remove or resuction the secretions.
- You may not be creating an adequate seal with your mouth, so:
  1. reposition your mouth and try mouth to mouth-and-nose again.
  2. try mouth-to-nose or mouth-to-mouth instead.
- You may not be providing strong enough breaths, so blow slightly harder.

The heart rate usually is abnormally slow (less than 100 beats per minute) with oxygen deprivation and increases with oxygen. If his heart rate remains less than 60 beats per minute even though air is moving adequately in and out of his chest, administer chest compressions at a rate of about 100 per minute (while administering the breaths) to maintain blood circulation. For each chest compression, using your fingers, press the lower half of his sternum down about one-third to one-half his anteroposterior diameter (the distance between his chest and the back) and release. Stop ventilation and compressions when he has spontaneous breaths and an adequate pulse.

All of these actions simply revive and stabilize the newborn. You should still take him to the hospital immediately.

Prevention and Preparation

Learn cardiopulmonary resuscitation (CPR) and take refresher courses. Pay as much attention to the sections on infants as the sections on adults. Although all the steps previously listed are general steps, definitely consult the latest American Heart Association Pediatric Advanced Life Support (PALS) course manual for details. The PALS guidelines are frequently changed in subtle or not-so-subtle ways. Check with your medical school or the American Heart Association to obtain the manual and take the certification course. Memorize the newborn CPR algorithms and techniques. Even if you don't become an obstetrician or a neonatologist, stay acquainted with childbirth procedures and complications. You never know when this knowledge will become useful—think of all the people you know, including your friends, family members, or you or your spouse, who might be pregnant.

If possible, don't deliver a baby alone. Other people can assist and call for help. Locate warm, dry blankets or the equivalent before the delivery. Keep the room warm and the mother as comfortable as possible. The mother (and you) should avoid sedatives. Most of all, keep everyone, including yourself, calm. Remember, even though the little one will have quite a challenging day, birth is a natural process and many newborns have successfully gone through similar circumstances.

Notes

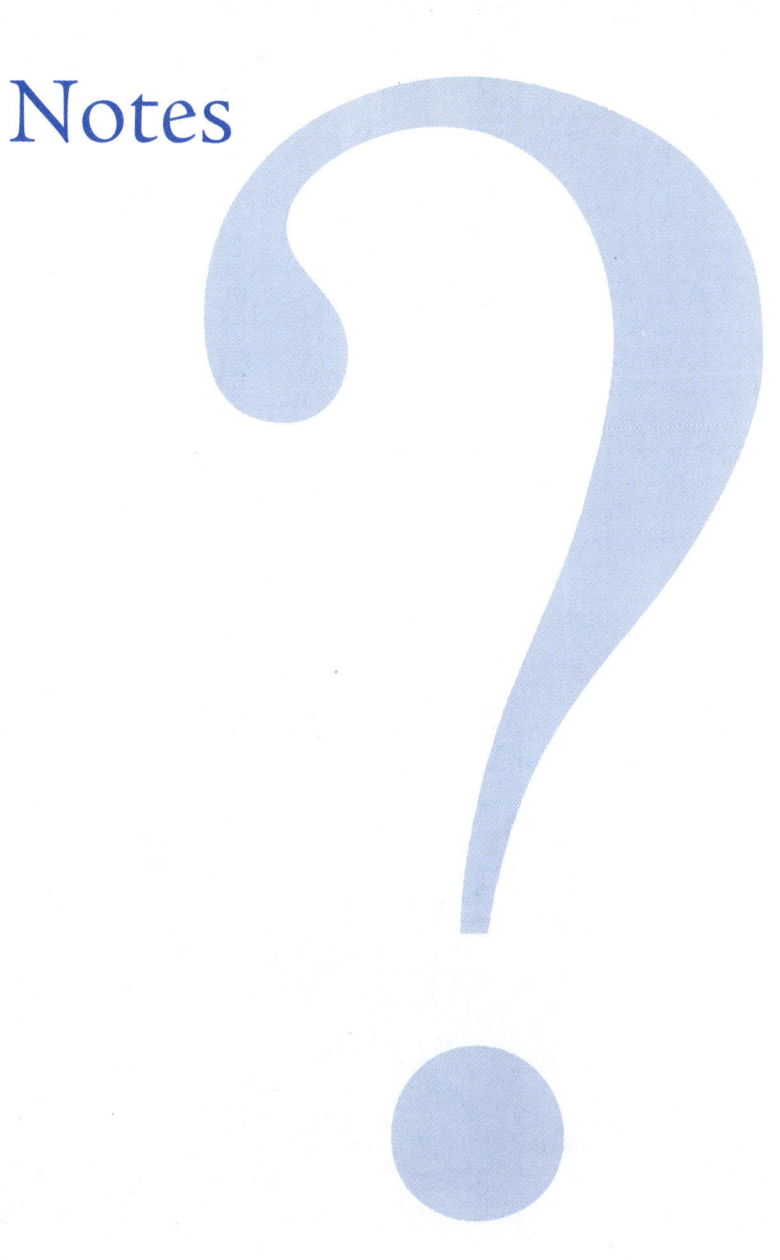

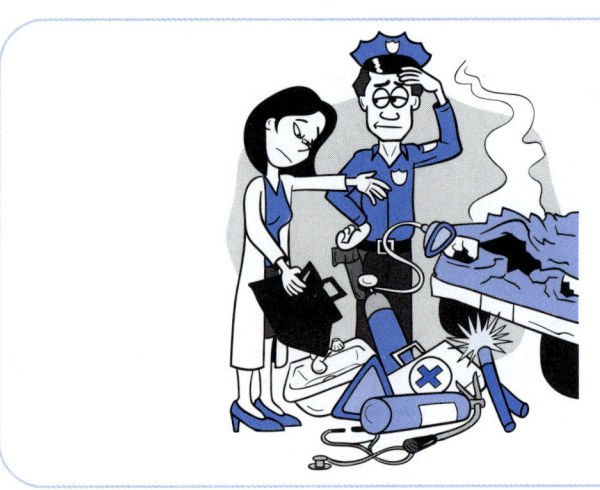

What if . . .

You're present at an automobile accident?

Automobile accidents are far too common and potentially extremely complicated situations. Ranging from simple fender-benders to the horrendous multicar pile-ups seen on television, car accidents can cause significant physical, emotional, legal, and financial damage. Cars can inflict nearly any kind of injury, external and obvious, or internal and insidious. Even long after the accident occurred, things can catch fire, poisonous chemicals can leak, objects can roll, and other vehicles can crash into an accident scene.

Bystanders can provide potentially life-saving assistance. Most states have Good Samaritan laws that protect assisting bystanders from being sued. However, even with good intentions, bystanders can also harm the victims and, as a result, not be protected. As a general rule, bystanders should make sure that by the time professional rescue personnel (police, firemen, and emergency medical transport personnel) arrive, victims are in better or at least the same condition as they found them.

What To Do

Your actions should depend on the severity of the accident and injuries, the location and conditions, the personnel available, and the timing of the accident and your arrival. Therefore, follow these steps:

- **Take a few moments to assess the situation.** Of course, a minor "fender-bender" won't require most of the following actions. Note the direction and location of traffic, objects or structures that may explode or collapse, and anything potentially hazardous. Keep yourself out of harm's way; you can't help anyone if you become incapacitated as well. Determine if professional rescue teams are already present. If so, offer assistance, but don't interfere. Obey the professionals as their training, experience, and understanding likely exceeds yours. Stay vigilant and warn them of developing situations (such as a neglected victim, leaking fuel, and oncoming traffic) that they might not notice. If no professionals are around, follow these steps:

- **Prevent additional accidents.** If you're in a motor vehicle, park it in a place that won't obstruct traffic and inhibit rescue personnel from reaching the victims. You or other bystanders should warn oncoming cars by turning on hazard lights, waving arms and flags, or setting up road flares to create a several hundred foot buffer zone around the accident. Don't put flares next to leaking gasoline. A visible buffer zone is especially important when visibility is low, victims are lying on the road, or the accident is located on a curve in the road. In the absence of flares or signs, consider positioning vehicles to create a protective barrier in a manner that's clearly visible to oncoming traffic.

- **Promptly call for emergency help (police, fire, and ambulance).** Never assume that others have made the calls. If you can't personally make the calls, ask as many bystanders or passing motorists as possible to do so to ensure that the call is actually made.

- **Unless absolutely necessary, don't move the victims.** Rescue professionals have the experience and equipment to move and remove victims without causing additional injury. Of course, if no professionals are available and the victim must be moved immediately to save her life (if, for example, the car is on fire), then you may have no choice. To be on the safe side, handle the victim as if she has neck and back injuries, as they're so common in automobile accidents, by supporting the neck and back, keeping them as immobile as possible.

- **Ask the victims if they need assistance.** Speaking to the victims will help determine their level of consciousness, the danger they may be in, and their desire for assistance. From their vantage point, they may be able to see and alert you about problems that aren't clearly visible (such as a fire, another victim, dripping gasoline, and unstable surfaces). Assisting someone who refuses to be assisted may make you liable for injuries you accidentally cause and disqualify you from being protected by Good Samaritan laws. So, when the victim declines assistance, if possible, wait for professional rescuers. Administer mouth-to-mouth or cardiopulmonary resuscitation (CPR) if the victim isn't breathing. If you aren't properly trained in CPR, find someone who is.

- **Protect the victims.** *Protect* doesn't mean *treat*. Don't administer first aid, such as bandaging or splinting injuries and administering medications. Be very conservative unless the victim is in immediate, life-threatening danger. Your goal should be to stabilize the situation until the professionals arrive. Reduce fire risk by removing highly flammable objects and turning off the motors of the cars involved in the accident, if possible. Keep the victim warm and shielded from the sun or rain to prevent shock. Encourage and reassure the victim. To stop profuse bleeding from easily accessible wounds, apply pressure with a clean cloth to stop the flow of blood. Be gentle if this wound is at a particularly vulnerable location like the head, neck or chest, as too much pressure may cause more injury.

- **Encourage victims and bystanders to remain until professionals arrive.** Victims and bystanders may be needed as witnesses. Most importantly, medical professionals should examine all victims for hidden internal injuries.

Prevention and Preparation

Although most people are aware of the behaviors that lead to car accidents (such as speeding; taking unnecessary risks; and driving while eating, drinking, impaired, or sleepy), many still continue these risky behaviors. In fact, medical students, physicians-in-training, and physicians commonly drive while sleepy. Curbing and encouraging others to curb such behaviors would certainly make the roads safer. Also, drive "defensively" and be prepared to handle other drivers' crazy behavior. Use seat belts at all times, install available safety features, and keep your car well-maintained.

Understand your state's Good Samaritan laws. Consider keeping the following items in your car: emergency road flares, warning triangles or cones, a flashlight with extra batteries, a thermal blanket, towels, bottled water, a tool kit, a first aid kit, and a fire extinguisher. Although storing these items may seem like a burden, you never know when they'll make a big difference.

What if . . .

A dinner guest is choking?

The most dangerous activity people do isn't bungee-jumping, skydiving, or car racing. Rather, it's something performed multiple times every day: eating. If we didn't need food to live, eating would be considered a health hazard. In addition to overeating, which can develop into obesity, eating can lead to severe allergic reactions, vomiting and diarrhea from poorly cooked food, or choking.

Choking occurs when food gets stuck in the throat or windpipe and it's more common than you might think. Because it's so common, restaurants are required to hang a poster that describes how you can help a choking victim. So, if you forget what you read in this *What if,* just remember to look for the poster. Be forewarned: this might happen to you, so pay attention.

Choking in adults is commonly caused by food, especially meat. Children, on the other hand, like to put nonfood items in their mouths, such as small toys, beads, or jewelry clasps. Things that people do *while* they eat may actually increase their risk of choking. Talking excitedly or laughing while chewing a piece of meat, eating too quickly, or walking or playing with food in the mouth may precipitate choking. Also, drinking alcohol while eating can dull the nerves that aid in swallowing and cause choking. We've all likely attempted at least one of these activities, perhaps even in combination, so it's a wonder that more people don't choke while eating.

What To Do

It's fairly easy to recognize when someone is choking because suddenly you'll notice an expression of terror or panic on his face. He may turn purple, start to gasp or wheeze, and clutch his throat. When a choking person attempts to cough, no sound is emitted because the windpipe is blocked by the food. The person may clutch his throat, the universal sign for choking. The treatment is the Heimlich maneuver, followed by cardiopulmonary resuscitation (CPR) if the person becomes unconscious from the lack of oxygen. The Heimlich increases intrathoracic pressure to force the object from the throat or windpipe.

Performing the Heimlich on Someone Else

Pull the choking victim to a standing position in front of you, wrap your arms around his waist, and bend him slightly forward. Make a fist with your dominant hand and place it slightly above the person's navel. Grasp your fist with your other hand and press hard into the upper abdomen with a quick upward thrust. Repeat this until the object is dislodged.

Performing the Heimlich on Yourself

Performing the Heimlich maneuver on yourself is challenging but necessary if you're alone. While leaning over a table or the back of your chair, position your fist slightly above your navel. Grasp your fist with your other hand and push inward and upward into the abdomen. Repeat this until the object is dislodged.

Performing the Heimlich on a Pregnant Woman

Women far along in their pregnancy deserve special mention because pushing on their protuberant abdomen may harm the baby. Proper positioning of your hands ensures the baby's safety. Position your fist just below the lowest ribs of her ribcage, at the base of her breastbone, above the abdomen. The maneuver itself is otherwise the same. You may also use this modified hand position for very obese people with large bellies.

Performing the Heimlich on an Infant

To perform the Heimlich on an infant, sit on a chair while holding the infant face down along your forearm that is resting on your thigh for extra support. With the heel of your hand, thump the infant in the middle of his back between

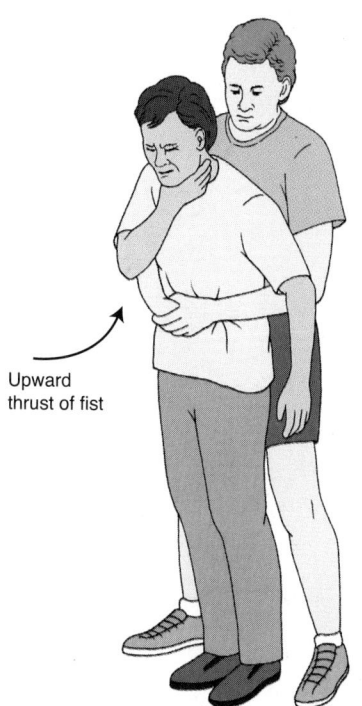

Upward
thrust of fist

Proper positioning for Heimlich maneuver.

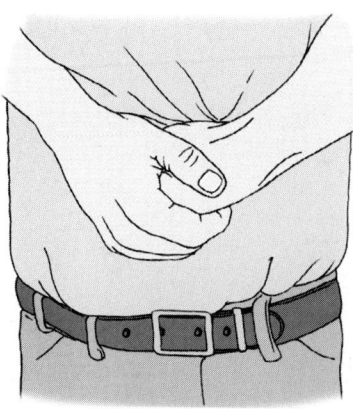

Position of hands for Heimlich maneuver on an adult.

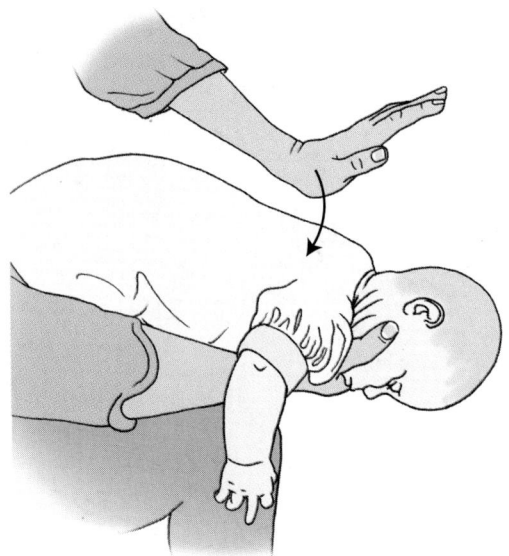

Step 1 of the Heimlich maneuver on an infant.

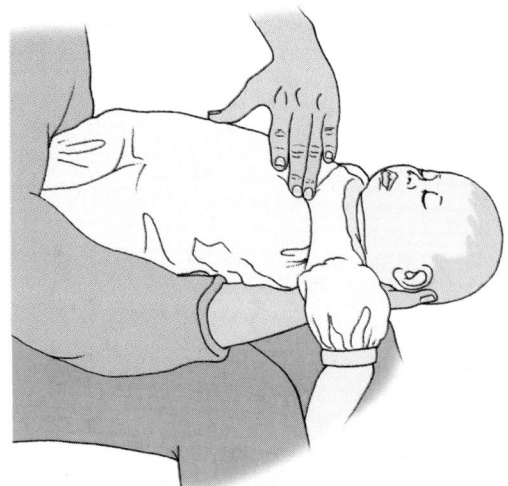

Step 2 of the Heimlich maneuver on an infant.

WATCH OUT FOR...

If the Heimlich Fails

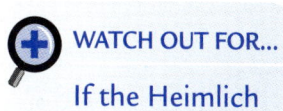

If a choking victim becomes unconscious or stops breathing when you're trying to deliver the Heimlich maneuver, position him on the ground, facing up. Open his mouth and sweep the back of the throat with your fingers to see if you can manually remove the obstruction. If you don't see or feel anything, resume the Heimlich by straddling the person, grasping your fist just above the navel, and thrusting upward and inward. After each thrust, open the mouth and sweep the throat to remove the obstruction. Repeat as necessary. If the patient doesn't resume breathing, have someone call 911 while you begin rescue breathing and CPR.

the shoulder blades firmly but gently five times. If the object doesn't become dislodged, turn the infant over so that he's face up on your forearm, with the head lower than the body. With two fingers, give five chest compressions on the center of the infant's breastbone. Repeat the entire cycle if needed.

Prevention and Preparation

There are plenty of ways you can prevent choking, especially in small children. Never leave small objects lying around (such as beads or small parts of toys that could fall off) and don't give foods like grapes, peanuts, popcorn, or big pieces of meat to small children. Try to resist the temptation to drink too much alcohol, eat too quickly, or talk or tell jokes with food in your mouth. Who knew that the adage "don't talk with your mouth full" actually has a scientific basis and that mom is right!

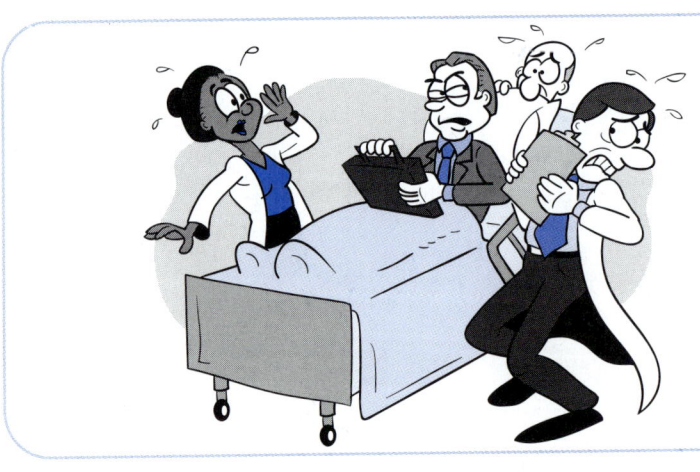

What if . . .

You need to help someone who's a lawyer?

"This is a 43-year-old female lawyer who presents with . . ." Have you ever heard this kind of presentation opening on rounds? Why do some physicians seem more on guard or wary when a patient is a lawyer, rather than a management consultant, an administrative assistant, a librarian, or a financial planner? Is it because certain viruses target lawyers? Do attorneys have tougher skin to penetrate with a catheter or needle? Are there environmental exposures that afflict attorneys and not others who work in similar office settings? Are lawyers actually a different species from humans?

Although some defendants in malpractice cases may claim that lawyers are a different species, basic taxonomy tells you that they aren't. With the staggering number and cost of malpractice lawsuits in this country, many physicians consciously or unconsciously associate lawyers with malpractice lawsuits and may assume that a lawyer is more likely to sue or know other lawyers who are willing to sue.

What To Do

Before you automatically assume that an attorney is carefully observing you and finding ways to sue you, remember that, just like physicians, there are a wide variety of personalities and job descriptions among lawyers. In fact "ambulance-chasing" malpractice or personal injury lawyers make up only a small percentage of the total number of lawyers. For their 2006 America's Best Graduate School rankings, *U.S. News and World Report* ranked 179 U.S. law schools. Think about how many graduates these law schools produce each year. Many specialize in a wide variety of nonmedical-related issues, including patents and trademarks, taxes, the environment, corporations, immigration, entertainment, and employment. A number of lawyers don't even practice law anymore, having entered politics, business, writing, entertainment (for example, Ben Stein from *Ferris Beuller's Day Off* and *Win Ben Stein's Money* is a lawyer), and even medicine.

Moreover, the fact is, anyone can bring a lawsuit against you. The person doesn't need to be a lawyer. He can be of any occupation, ethnicity, gender, socioeconomic status, or background. He can even be a physician. You can't predict who will be more or less likely to use legal action. Lawsuits arise from several different situations. In some cases, legitimate negligence occurred. In others, the physician made an honest, human mistake. In still others, bad outcomes occurred despite the fact that everything was done correctly and properly. Sometimes, no bad outcomes or mistakes occurred. The plaintiff may simply have a personal dislike for or vendetta against the physician or be looking to exploit the system to make money. As you can see, these situations can occur with anyone.

Finally, some of the patients who don't reveal their professions may in fact be attorneys. Either no one asked them their occupations or they chose not to reveal it because they were no longer practicing, weren't in a condition to answer, or didn't want to be treated differently. In fact, if they're looking for lawsuits, it's possible that they may want to catch health-care workers off guard by "hiding" as a non-attorney. What's more, patients who aren't attorneys may have spouses, siblings, parents, children, or best friends who are attorneys. The bottom line is that lawyers can be anywhere, they aren't necessarily more likely to sue you, and lawsuits can come from anyone. Therefore, in this case, "occupational profiling" isn't going to help you.

Therefore, there is little attorney-specific advice. The patient's occupation shouldn't determine whether or how you treat the patient. You must be vigilant, conscientious, and careful with every patient. If possible, try to develop a rapport with each patient and communicate well. Carefully document what you do. Act naturally. If you keep thinking that this patient is an attorney, then you may act nervous or uncomfortable, which may unnecessarily worry the patient or make him wonder what you have to hide. Don't treat the patient any differently. Don't do any procedures that you aren't qualified to do or comfortable doing. Recognize situations where supervision or accompaniment by another health-care worker or witness is important, such as during breast or pelvic examinations or anything associated with risk or discomfort.

Prevention and Preparation

Properly learn and practice procedures. Sharpen your patient interaction and communication skills. Learn what must be documented and how to document it. Physicians and physicians-in-training should make an effort to understand the medical legal system as well as they can. Nowadays, learning the legal ram-

RESOURCES

Information on medical-legal issues is available from physicians, lawyers, physician-lawyers (or lawyer-physicians), and hospitals.

Physicians
Most major physician societies have sections on legal issues on their websites. For example, the American Medical Association website *(www.ama-assn.org)* has a "Legal issues for physicians" section under "Professional Resources."

Lawyers
The American Bar Association *(www.abanet.org)* has a Health Law Section, which has a number of publications and courses. Although many of these are geared toward lawyers, it can be helpful to see what the "other side" is writing and thinking.

Physician-Lawyers
The American College of Legal Medicine *(www.aclm.org)* publishes two newsletters, *Legal Medicine Perspectives* and *Legal Medicine Q&A,* to keep physicians current on medical-legal developments and concerns. They also publish a textbook, *Legal Medicine,* which reviews the legal implications of medical practice.

Hospitals
Many hospitals and medical centers have Risk Management Departments that specialize in protecting the medical center from legal problems and providing information on medical-legal issues to physicians. They likely have pamphlets and handbooks on important issues. Many have websites.

ifications of what you do may be just as important as knowing histology and pharmacology. Ask experienced physicians about important legal issues and concerns. Understand important medical-legal decisions, cases, and policies. In the end, you're better off paying more attention to the law and what you're doing than whether or not your patient is a lawyer.

What if . . .

You're asked to use an AED in an airplane or other public place?

Automatic external defibrillators (AEDs) are increasingly available on airplanes and in many public places for use in prompt treatment of cardiac arrest due to ventricular fibrillation (VFib). VFib occurs when thousands of cardiac muscle cells contract randomly in an utterly chaotic, ineffective pattern. During VFib, the ventricles stop pumping and death quickly ensues.

The most common cause of VFib is a myocardial infarction in progress. However, many other structural and acquired heart diseases may cause VFib. Vfib in marathon runners is often noted; however, the risk of VFib in these athletes is much lower than in the general population, although higher than in other types of exercise. Autopsies of these marathon runners commonly reveal previously undiagnosed heart disease. Another cause of Vfib in athletes is direct trauma to the precordium, such as with a baseball, helmet, or hockey puck. VFib can also result from electrolyte disorders or an unknown cause.

VFib causes approximately two-thirds of all cardiac arrest cases. For every minute that a person experiences VFib without undergoing defibrillation, chances of survival decrease by 10%. Thus, use of an AED has caused dramatic improvement in the treatment of extra-hospital cardiac arrest. In fact, many physicians and experts in prehospital emergency care believe that using the AED takes precedence over starting basic CPR. According to an almost 2-year-long study conducted by the National Heart, Lung, and Blood Institute (NHLBI) and the American Heart Association (AHA), victims of cardiac arrest were almost twice as likely to survive when treated with CPR and an AED than those victims treated with CPR alone.

Even so, if access to an AED is delayed, you should immediately begin CPR. The mechanical chest compressions and ventilation procedures of basic CPR will provide minimal circulation to vital organs until an AED or other form of defibrillator is available.

What To Do

When you're alerted to a cardiac arrest, send someone to call for help. When you've established that the victim is unable to be aroused and is pulseless, turn on the AED by opening the case or pushing the large ON/OFF button (depending on the manufacturer of the machine). When the device is turned on, audible, computer-generated instructions explain what to do. The automated voice should prompt you to place the two thin, circular pads supplied with the AED on the bare skin of the victim's chest. Place one pad on the right side of the chest, superior to the nipple and inferior to the clavicle. Place the other pad on the left side of the person, inferior to the left breast. In female patients it's usually unnecessary to remove the patient's bra.

WARNING! If the patient has a permanent pacemaker, don't place the pad over the pacemaker generator. Delivering electrical countershock to the generator could disable it. The pacemaker's generator will be visible and palpable as a solid, circular, subcutaneous mass on the anterior surface of the chest. Look for it when you're placing the pads.

Most AEDs have a SHOCK button that must be pushed to deliver the defibrillating electrical energy. The device determines whether the person is in VFib before it actually attempts defibrillation. The AED then instructs you to "Stand clear and push the shock button." Stand clear of the patient and activate the AED's electrical discharge by pushing the SHOCK button. The device delivers an electrical charge across the precordium, causing the myocardium to completely depolarize and briefly stop all activity, including the Vfib.

If all goes well, the heart then restarts with a normal electrical impulse from the sinoatrial node, yielding normal sinus rhythm (NSR). If NSR doesn't follow, the AED reanalyzes the heart rhythm to see if further defibrillation is needed.

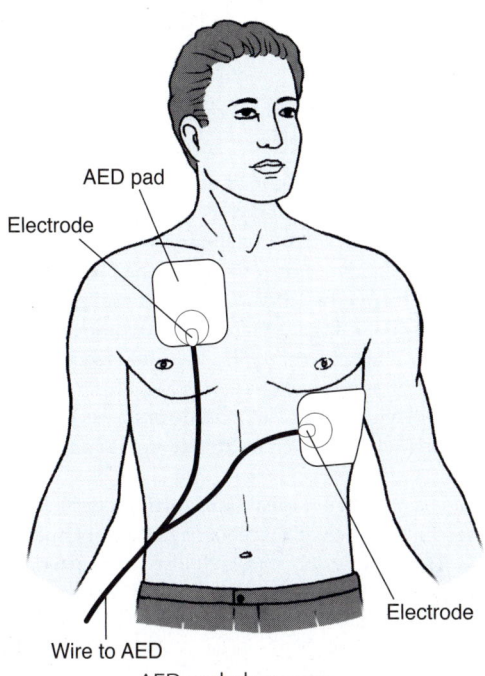

AED pad

Electrode

Electrode

Wire to AED

AED pad placement.

Prevention and Preparation

As someone with a medical background, you may feel compelled to take action or be asked to use an AED to help a victim of cardiac arrest. If you haven't received training on the proper use of an AED, you can obtain it from local chapters of the AHA. The *AHA Heartsaver AED Manual* is an excellent resource. Websites that can also help include:

- AHA at *http://www.americanheart.org*
- American College of Emergency Physicians at *http://www.acep.org*
- Call, Clear, and Shock, Inc., at *http://www.defib.org* (a company that offers AEDs, related products, and education).

Although the AED is designed for ease of use, previous experience and training can give this *What if* a lifesaving outcome.

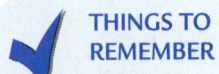

THINGS TO REMEMBER

When you use an AED

If someone says he or she has been trained on the proper use of an AED, you may want to let the person perform the procedure while you watch the patient closely. Remember to have someone call 9-1-1 or summon additional help.

In an airplane, ask the flight attendant to inform the pilot of the circumstances. Because cabin pressure has a direct impact on the partial pressure of oxygen in the blood, request that the pilot bring the plane to an altitude at which the cabin pressure is approximately what it is at sea level (typically 22,000 feet) and then to the nearest, safe-landing airport that has emergency services available. (Commercial airlines maintain cabin pressure equivalent to an altitude of about 8000 feet, which reduces atmospheric partial pressure of oxygen by 25% compared to partial pressure at sea level.)

Remember to start basic CPR if normal sinus rhythm doesn't resume or repeated shocks are unsuccessful and the patient remains pulseless. Usually, the AED will prompt you to check for a pulse and start CPR after three attempts at defibrillation. If the patient responds, comfort the patient but don't remove the pads. You may need to defibrillate again before more help arrives.

What if ...

You encounter an unanticipated allergic reaction?

Allergic reactions are caused by an overactive immune system and can present a range of symptoms, from an annoying pruritic skin rash (urticaria) or rhinorrhea to acute, life-threatening upper airway edema with laryngeal obstruction (anaphylaxis). Although these reactions are mediated by various pathophysiological mechanisms, as shown in the table, they're all immune-mediated (mainly by IgE) and imply some prior exposure to the responsible antigen. In short, when the antigen enters the body, it binds to IgE, which crosslinks with IgE membrane receptors on mast cells and basophils, releasing stored chemical mediators that wreak havoc on the rest of the body. A similar reaction to anaphylaxis is an *anaphylactoid reaction,* which isn't IgE mediated but manifests very similar symptoms. Common instigators are radiopaque contrast media and medications (such as aspirin).

Anaphylaxis, thought to occur in less than 1% of the population, rarely causes death and usually lacks a causative agent. Of the identifiable etiologies, food (such as peanuts and shellfish) is probably the most common cause, followed by insect stings (*Hymenoptera*), antibiotics, aspirin, and latex. Those con-

● HYPERSENSITIVITY CLASSIFICATIONS

The table below lists the different types of hypersensitivity reactions along with an example and the mediators for each.

Hypersensitivity Reactions	Examples	Mediators
Type I (immediate hypersensitivity)	Food allergies, insect bites, drug allergies	IgE
Type II (cytotoxic)	Immune globulin transfusion reactions	IgG or IgM
Type III (immune complex)	Blood transfusion reactions	IgG or IgM-complex
Type IV (delayed hypersensitivity)	Poison ivy rash	T cell

sidered at risk for severe reactions usually have predisposing atopy.

The initial immediate reaction usually involves the skin, with generalized warmth, tingling, and intense itching. These symptoms may be followed by cough, chest tightness, hoarseness, lightheadedness, and abdominal cramping. Rapid progression to severe, life-threatening reactions may occur, including myocardial ischemia, pulmonary edema, angioedema, laryngeal obstruction, and complete cardiovascular collapse. Most reactions occur immediately—within seconds to minutes after exposure to the triggering antigen, and may rapidly progress from mild urticaria to shock or respiratory compromise within 30 minutes. The duration of symptoms is variable; the reaction may be promptly terminated or last up to 2 days with treatment.

 WATCH OUT FOR...

Latex

Latex allergies, caused by latex gloves, have recently become a serious health hazard for health-care providers, patients, and rubber industry workers. Latex condoms are another potential cause, but alternative natural skin and polyurethane condoms are readily available. Although the most common symptoms are urticaria, rhinitis, and occupational asthma, true anaphylaxis may occur. Treatment follows the guidelines outlined in the text.

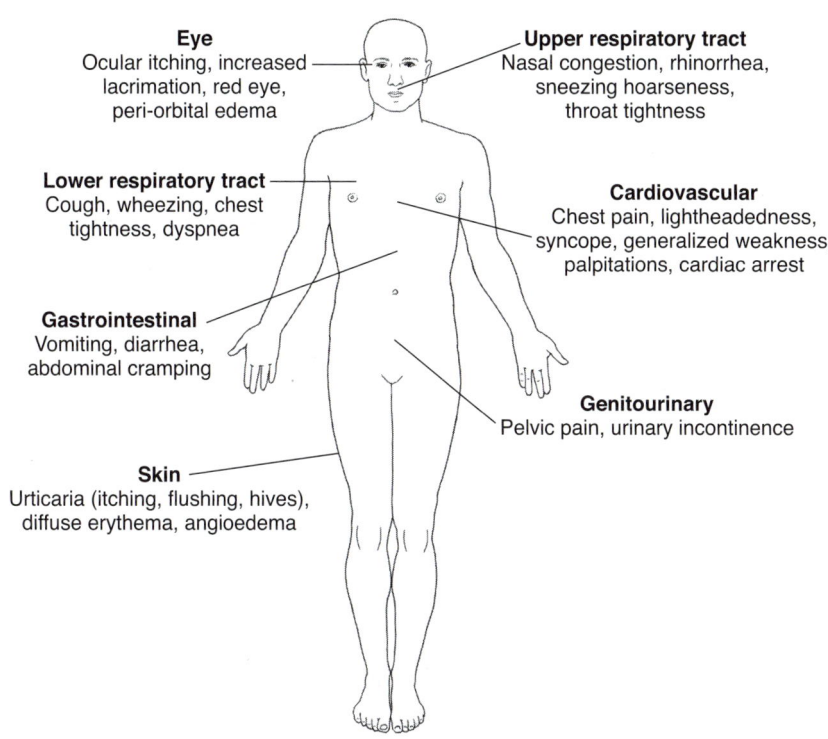

Eye
Ocular itching, increased lacrimation, red eye, peri-orbital edema

Upper respiratory tract
Nasal congestion, rhinorrhea, sneezing hoarseness, throat tightness

Lower respiratory tract
Cough, wheezing, chest tightness, dyspnea

Cardiovascular
Chest pain, lightheadedness, syncope, generalized weakness, palpitations, cardiac arrest

Gastrointestinal
Vomiting, diarrhea, abdominal cramping

Genitourinary
Pelvic pain, urinary incontinence

Skin
Urticaria (itching, flushing, hives), diffuse erythema, angioedema

Signs and symptoms of anaphylaxis.

What To Do

Your course of action depends on the type of allergic reaction:

- *Previously recognized allergies:* Typically, people with known severe allergic reactions will be prescribed an injectable form of epinephrine (EpiPen) to use in the event of an inadvertent exposure. This should be promptly injected into the deltoid or thigh at the earliest sign of the allergic reaction to prevent progression of symptoms.
- *Localized reaction:* Insect stings or contact with tree or plant oils and metal alloys in jewelry cause localized skin reactions. These generally cause pruritus and swelling at the site of contact, but, in the case of insect stings, may progress to airway edema and bronchospasm.

Local measures, such as dependent positioning of the extremity,
removing the stinger, or cooling with ice to locally vasoconstrict the site of exposure can decrease antigen absorption. Oral antihistamines may further decrease the local reaction. The most commonly used antihistamine is diphenhydramine hydrochloride (Benadryl) 25 to 50 mg every 4 to 6 hours taken orally.

- *Systemic reaction:* People with moderate to severe reactions (such as hoarseness, vomiting, tongue or lip swelling, and chest tightness) should be taken to the Emergency Department immediately for treatment with parenteral medications. Useful temporizing measures include administration of epinephrine (if available), Benadryl 50 mg, and two puffs of an albuterol inhaler. Albuterol may alleviate the bronchospasm and wheezing.

THINGS TO REMEMBER

When you encounter anaphylaxis

- Even though urticaria is the most common symptom of anaphylaxis, respiratory and cardiovascular collapse may occur without skin manifestations.
- Mild symptoms should be treated aggressively to prevent progression to severe anaphylaxis and airway compromise.
- Epinephrine is the immediate drug of choice for anaphylaxis and should be carried by those with known severe allergies.

Prevention and Preparation

Avoidance of the antigen is the best strategy to prevent anaphylaxis, however, inadvertent exposure to allergens is unavoidable. People with severe bee allergies should avoid contact and try to carry an EpiPen with them (easier said than done, due to expiration dates and temperature considerations). Careful, serious questioning of restaurant personnel regarding the use of nuts (especially peanuts) in their cooking can save a life.

Notes

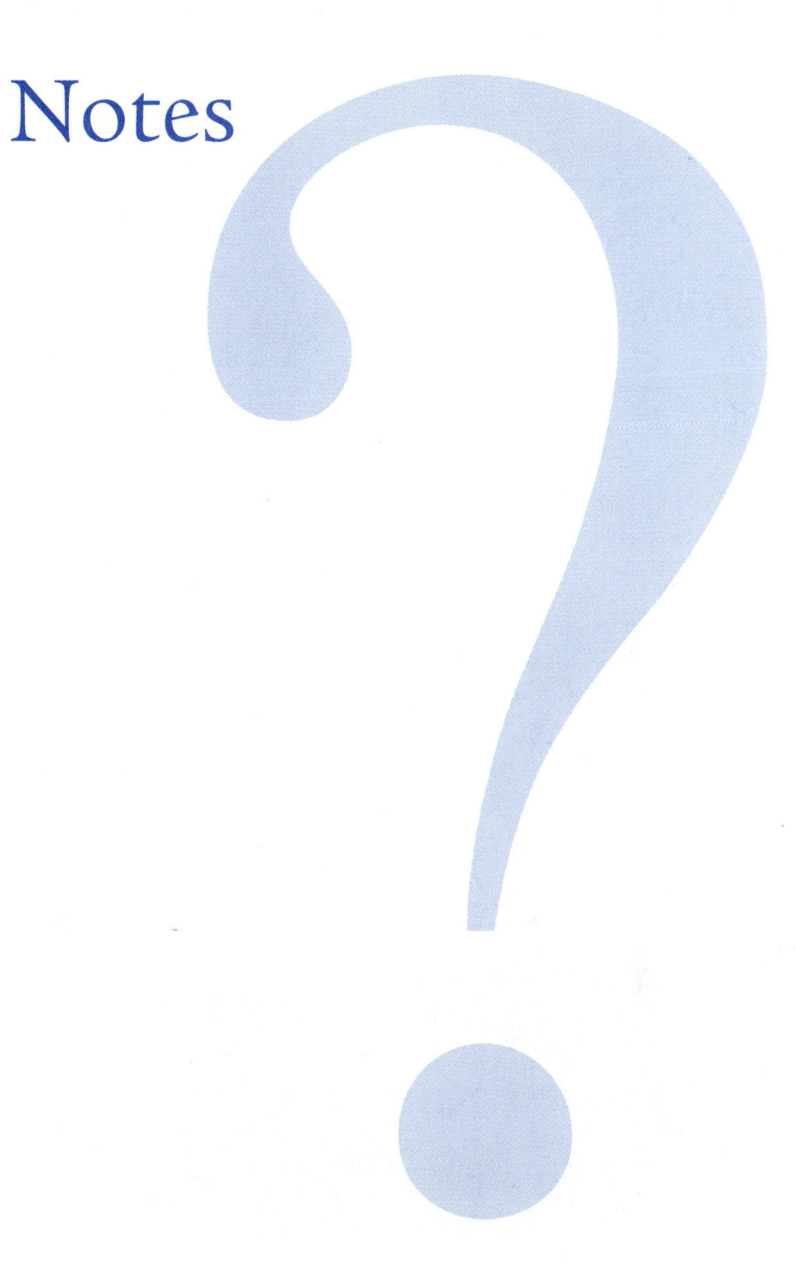

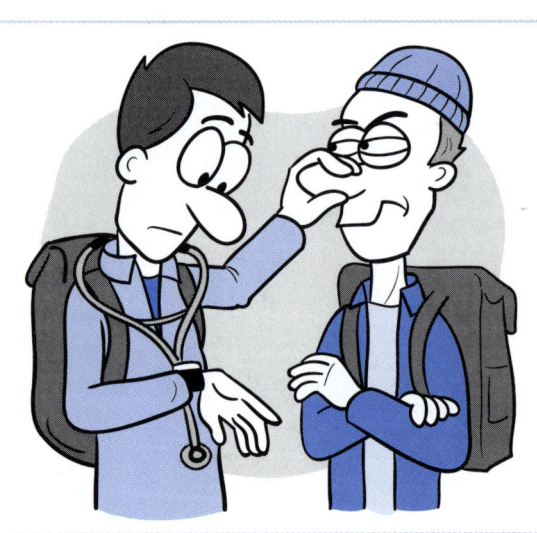

What if . . .

Your companion has a nosebleed that won't stop?

Bleeding from anywhere on the body can be frightening. A nosebleed (epistaxis), although seldom life-threatening, is easily noticeable by others, which can lead to further embarrassment and anxiety. Epistaxis occurs when the blood vessels in the nose are disrupted and, because the vessels are all arterial, they can cause profuse bleeding. Bleeding from vessels located in the anterior-inferior nasal septum, known as *Kiesselbach's plexus,* causes most epistaxis and is easily controlled by pinching the nose. In contrast, bleeding from the back of the nose is rare but more difficult to control, because it's hard to reach the back of the nose to stop the bleeding.

The most common cause of epistaxis, which may be fairly obvious, is facial trauma, such as getting punched in the nose during a fight or getting elbowed in the face during a high-energy basketball game. Interestingly, the most common nose trauma is actually self-induced: nose picking. All people, kids and adults included, have picked their noses at some point in time. Another cause is respiratory infections. People with colds blow their noses frequently and usually with enough force to cause some bleeding. This type of bleeding happens even more frequently in winter months when low humidity dries out the nasal mucosa, making it easily friable. Moreover, there are some people who simply bleed more easily than others—for example, those taking anticoagulants such as warfarin, or antiplatelet medications such as aspirin, or those with clotting deficiencies such as hemophiliacs.

What To Do

Ask the patient to blow his nose to clear any blood clots. Then apply pressure on the nasal septum by pinching both sides of the nose, compressing the cartilaginous part of the nose, for 20 minutes. Make sure you use a clock to time this step accurately because 5 minutes of nose pinching may feel like an eternity of discomfort. An adequate, though unattractive alternative is clamping a clothespin across the nose. Resist the temptation to tilt the head backward because blood that drips down the back of the throat could choke the patient. Keep the patient in an upright position, if possible. If the bleeding is massive or persistent, continue to apply pressure but immediately bring the patient to the hospital for definitive treatment, such as nasal packing or cautery.

If you're far from a medical facility and applying pressure isn't helping, you may attempt to moderate the bleeding by packing the nose with a regular vaginal tampon, if available. Packing the tampon supplies constant, firm pressure against the blood vessels in the nose to stop the bleeding. Remove the tampon from the applicator and insert it directly and quickly (with a gentle but firm pressure) into the nostril that appears to be the origin of the bleeding, aiming directly toward the back of the head (occiput). The string attached to the tampon should be taped to the cheek so that it doesn't break off. It will eventually be used to pull out the packing. If you feel the need to use a tampon in each nostril, make sure the patient can breath adequately through his mouth.

WARNING!!! Patients at high risk for potentially life-threatening epistaxis should proceed as quickly as possible to a hospital for additional treatment. Patients in this high-risk category include the very elderly, patients on anticoagulants, and patients with bleeding disorders. Other signs and symptoms that should cause you to get the epistaxis patient to a hospital include chest pain, lightheadedness, syncope, shortness of breath, and choking from blood pouring down the pharynx (suggesting posterior epistaxis).

Prevention and Preparation

Unless you plan to wear a helmet every time you leave the house, the only nasal trauma you can prevent is self-induced trauma. Stop picking your nose and avoid blowing your nose too hard when you catch a cold. In the winter time, using a humidifier at home or coating the inside of your nose with a thin layer of Vaseline can prevent the mucosa from drying out and becoming easily friable. When faced with the unexpected nosebleed, remember that your most useful tool is your hand or a simple clothespin. Most nosebleeds can be stopped with pressure applied in the right spot on the nose. Knowing that you can stop most epistaxis with pressure (pinching) and patience, prepares you well for this *What if* scenario.

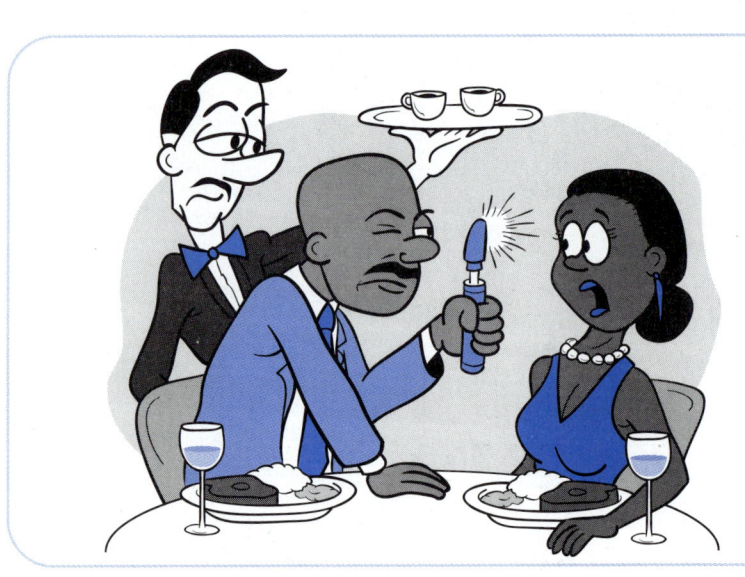

What if . . .

Your friend has a foreign body in the eye?

Your first date with the person sitting across the dinner table is going well. You're enjoying your date's company, conversation flows effortlessly, and you're wondering if your companion might be the *one,* someone with whom you could develop a long-term relationship. All you need is one final sign that this person is the right person for you. Then you see something in your date's eye...

No, it isn't a sparkle, a glimmer, or a sign . . . It's a foreign body. Something is in the person's eye. Chances are you can't see the foreign body because it's usually a very small particle of wood, metal, hair, dust, glass, or fabric. Instead, you likely see the signs and symptoms of a foreign body, such as eye irritation, itching, burning, soreness, grittiness, and redness. Your date may be experiencing tearing, light sensitivity, decreased vision, or difficulty opening the eye. The irritation may be mild or intense, periodic, or continuous. The foreign body may be stuck on the cornea, conjunctiva, or under the eyelid, or may have penetrated the eye tissue. Symptoms don't always reliably indicate the severity of the problem because penetrating foreign bodies may be less painful than superficial ones. Moreover, the location of the irritation may not correspond to the location of the object.

WARNING!!! Although superficial foreign bodies usually aren't serious, penetrating ones can cause major injury and even loss of vision. However, superficial foreign bodies may also damage the eye or lead to infection, especially when not removed fairly soon. Moreover, superficial foreign bodies may eventually penetrate the eye. Bleeding, corneal abrasions, retinal damage, and cataracts are other possible complications of foreign bodies.

What To Do

Keep the person from rubbing or touching the eye. Have the person keep the eye shut as much as possible and avoid blinking. Unless your dinner engagement is in an ophthalmologist's office or an emergency department and you're properly trained, don't try to remove the object with your fingers or any other object, such as a matchstick, toothpick, or cotton swab. Moving or manipulating the eye may push the object deeper, causing more injury and making it more difficult to remove.

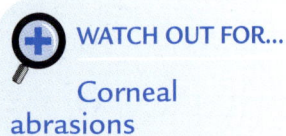

WATCH OUT FOR...

Corneal abrasions

Naturally, the emergency department or an eye clinic is better equipped to deal with corneal abrasions. The physician will usually apply topical anesthetic drops to numb the patient's cornea before examining the patient's eyes. The emergency department and clinic has access to such devices as slit lamps, eye charts, and imaging and surgical equipment to thoroughly inspect the eye, measure visual acuity, and remove the object. In addition, the physician will commonly perform a fluorescein examination to find any corneal abrasions caused by the foreign body.

If the foreign body is superficial, shutting the eyes will usually make the person produce tears, which commonly is enough to wash out the object. If this method doesn't work, try to find warm, clean water to gently rinse the person's eye. Because patients commonly have difficulty thoroughly rinsing their own eyes, you may have to assist the patient by turning the head or moving the water source back and forth. If there is any possibility that the object or object fragments remain in the person's eye after irrigation, contain toxic chemicals, or are unusually hot or cold, the person should be taken to the emergency department.

Your date's recent history may provide clues about what may be in her eye. For example, your date using a jackhammer prior to or during your dinner appointment would raise the likelihood of a penetrating eye injury. Activities, such as hammering, grinding, and chopping, in which sharp objects may be moving at high velocities raise the suspicion of a penetrating foreign body. Again, symptoms (or the absence of symptoms) can be misleading. If there is any concern that the object may be penetrating, don't try to remove it; instead, seek emergency department care immediately.

Prevention and Preparation

There are many ways you (or your date) can prevent foreign bodies from entering the eye. Although it may inhibit your vision, feel cumbersome, or look unattractive, protective eyewear should be worn whenever there is the risk of flying objects. Proper eyewear should shield the eyes not only in front but also on the sides as flying objects can come at any angle. Before touching anyone's eyes, wash your hands. In general, avoid rubbing your eyes. Foreign bodies can stick to your hands or other objects. Keep your contact lenses clean and change them in clean, relatively dustless surroundings.

In situations where flying objects are likely, have access to bottles of saline solution or clean eye baths. Don't dismiss minor irritations when foreign bodies are possible and promptly address the problem. This rule holds true especially if your date appears to be weeping excessively. It may not necessarily be the result of her feelings about you . . .

What if . . .

One-on-One Encounters

What if . . .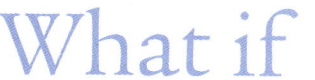

A patient makes a sexual advance toward you?

You'll definitely experience or suspect that a patient is making a sexual advance toward you in some form at least once during your career.

What To Do

Ethical behavior must prevail! You shouldn't pursue an advance toward you, even if you and the patient are single. It's entirely unethical to develop such a relationship with a patient or former patient.

Unless you're a psychiatrist, it's likely that you haven't had formal training for this situation. Here are some questions to ask yourself:

- Is this really what it seems? Is this the patient's actions or is it your feelings?
- Review what actually happened. Was it an explicit request or solicitation? Or was it a flirtatious comment or look? Or is it something you have said or done?
- Did the patient cross a boundary such as repeatedly touching you on the arm as he or she spoke with you about symptoms or problems?
- Does the patient usually dress provocatively for your visits?

- Have you crossed a boundary that you shouldn't, such as complimenting or commenting on the patient's clothing or manner of dress, talking about your personal problems, meeting the patient outside the usual clinical setting, or encouraging the use of your first name?

Answering "yes" to any of these questions can indicate inappropriate behavior and even a mild or severe psychological disorder (in the patient *or* doctor). Some of these actions can be symptoms of a specific psychological disorder, such as histrionic personality disorder. Other actions may be the products of a psychological response to the normal close interaction that occurs as a clinician takes care of a patient—for example, transference and countertransference.

In either case, it's important to reestablish the boundaries of the patient-physician relationship and do so without alienating the patient. Gently remind the patient that you're most able to help as a clinician and that is the limit of the relationship. Patients who fail to respond to your attempts to reestablish proper boundaries for the patient-physician relationship need additional psychological evaluation and counseling.

If you find that you're often having inappropriate feelings toward patients, you need professional help. There should be nothing provocative about a clinical examination. Stop seeing patients until you can get help. If it isn't possible to stop seeing patients while seeking help, be sure to always have a chaperone of the same sex of the patient in the examination room with you.

PSYCHOLOGICAL FACTORS

Here are two psychological factors that may play a part in inappropriate sexual behavior on the part of the patient or doctor.

Histrionic personality disorder

Histrionic personality disorder is defined in the *Diagnostic and Statistical Manual of Mental Disorders (DSM-IV)* as a pervasive pattern of excessive emotionality and attention seeking, beginning by early childhood and present in a variety of contexts, as indicated by five or more of the following:

- The person is uncomfortable in situations in which he or she isn't the center of attention.
- Interaction with others is often characterized by inappropriate sexually seductive behavior.
- The person displays rapidly shifting and shallow expression of emotions.
- The person consistently uses physical appearance to attract attention.
- The person has a style of speech that is excessively

impressionistic and lacking in detail.

- The person shows self-dramatization, theatricality, and exaggerated expression of emotion.
- The person is suggestible.
- The person considers relationships to be more intimate than they actually are.

Transference and countertransference

In brief, transference is a psychological phenomenon in which a patient sees the clinician as a significant person from his or her past and essentially "transfers" feelings about that person to the present situation. Transference happens in our day-to-day lives as well and is usually a subconscious response. Therefore, the clinician can experience this response toward the patient as well. When the clinician experiences this phenomenon, it's called *countertransference*. Psychiatrists have learned to recognize these phenomena in the patient-physician relationship and use them effectively in the course of psychotherapy.

Prevention and Preparation

In general, when you meet a patient for the first time and during all subsequent encounters, remember that you aren't trying to be a friend or companion to the person. You're trying to be their physician—a physician they can trust and respect. You should actively avoid crossing the boundaries previously described. For example, helping a young female patient with her coat sends an inappropriate message, unless she is so disabled that she needs your assistance *as a health-care professional*.

Self-awareness is crucial. If you find you're often having inappropriate feelings toward patients, seek professional help. Your state's medical society should have a program for physicians with behavioral problems or can refer you to a program. More than ever, referrals to these extremely helpful programs are sought by medical students and residents. Identifying these resources in advance and learning common methods to deal with these problems will help you successfully avoid or deal with this *What if* situation.

What if . . .

A patient of the opposite sex doesn't want you in the exam room?

This scenario is more common today than a decade ago. It's more likely to happen to you as a student and can be provoked by your own behavior or perceived discomfort. It's important to remember that one of the most important patient rights is the right to refuse medical care or portions of it, such as treatment and even diagnosis. Nevertheless, it's also important to make sure that patients are informed enough to make rational decisions about these matters.

What To Do

When a patient refuses to let you examine him or her, first, introduce or reintroduce yourself. Explain to the patient who you are and why you're in the room (your specific role). In order to have this further conversation with the patient, you may have to acknowledge that first refusal with a nonthreatening reply designed to put the patient at ease. An example of such a reply would be, "That won't be a problem, sir [madame] but, before the exam, I'll need to ask you a few questions and try to answer your questions." This brief explanation will usually give you the opportunity to determine the chief complaint and start taking a medical history of the present illness. More than half of the work of making a diagnosis is obtaining a good medical history and the data gleaned from such an interview is commonly far more useful than the physical examination.

In the process of taking the history, you have the opportunity to establish rapport with the patient. Make good use of that opportunity. First, avoid appearing defensive, condescending, or insulted by the patient's initial objection; doing so would only make matters worse. In addition, a more "patient-centered" approach to the medical interview, rather than the more tradition "doctor-centered" approach, can establish rapport and provide good clinical information about the patient.

Patient Central

The patient-centered approach usually begins with an introduction similar to the one just mentioned, during which you should introduce yourself and express your desire to ask questions. It's important to invite the patient to decide what he or she would like to talk about first. As the patient begins to discuss his or her concerns, be open and encourage verbal and nonverbal cues. Examples of encouraging cues are saying "uh-huh," "yes," or "I understand" or simply nodding your head. Eventually you'll be able to elicit symptoms and pursue them with clarifying questions, such as "When did that begin?" and "What seems to bring it on?" and "Is there anything you do that relieves it?" (in other words, eventually shifting over to the more doctor-centered approach).

Using this approach may bring you to a point where it's easy to accomplish a focused examination of the affected body part. For example, if you feel you've established adequate rapport, you might ask, "May I take a look at the arm that is painful?" Depending on the care setting or situation, such as an outpatient clinic or walk-in clinic, a focused examination may be all that is necessary to diagnose the problem. In the inpatient setting, someone will need to conduct a complete physical examination. If you've established good rapport with the patient, he or she may spontaneously tell you to do a more complete examination. If the patient doesn't verbalize this change of heart, make sure you've obtained as much information as you can, and then tell the patient you'll arrange for someone

> ### PATIENT-CENTERED INTERVIEWING
>
> For more complete information on the patient-centered interview and related techniques, see:
>
> - *The Patient's Story: Integrated Patient-Doctor Interviewing* by Robert C. Smith, MD. Little, Brown and Company, Boston, 1996.
> - *Patient-Centered Medicine: Transforming the Clinical Method* by Moira Stewart, et al. Radcliffe Publishing, Oxford, 2003.

of the same sex as the patient to come and perform the examination. Commonly such an offer at this point in the interview will prompt the patient to grant you permission to proceed with a more complete examination.

Prevention and Preparation

"Emotional intelligence" is a common phrase used to express how well you know and control yourself. Knowing yourself, your feelings, and your reactions in certain situations can help you help your patients get comfortable with you. Emotional intelligence gives you the best opportunity to help your patients by showing them your professionalism and your ability to diagnose and treat them, regardless of what sex you are. The patient wants a doctor, so act like one, look like one, and be one!

What if . . .

You have to give a patient bad news?

As medical students we were never taught how to tell a patient they have a terminal illness or cancer. It apparently was assumed that we would learn this through the legendary "Watch one, do one, teach one" process. People seek careers in the health professions to make diagnoses and provide remedies, and not for the opportunity to deliver bad news. It's always difficult to convey bad news. Although you shouldn't encounter this *What if* situation as a student, it will most probably occur during your postgraduate training period. The lack of training for this situation should cause most clinicians to want to prepare in advance.

What To Do

Giving a patient a cancer diagnosis is very difficult. The challenge in this instance is providing clear, accurate information and the appropriate hope for recovery. There are hundreds of cancers and, even within a specific cell-type, tremendous variation in prognosis and outcome.

Discuss the diagnosis with the patient in a room with privacy. Be clear and specific. We have seen far too many patients listen to their doctors discuss tumors or malignancies, only to have the patient later state, "At least it isn't cancer." So, be specific and try to describe the next steps in treatment and what to expect along the way. Provide the patient with plenty of opportunity to ask questions.

Difficult Diagnosis

In most instances, the diagnosis is made early enough that it's relatively easy to be optimistic and instill great hope for recovery. However, in some instances, the diagnosis comes late, metastases are present, or there has been a recurrence after initial treatment. In these circumstances, it isn't as easy to instill hope, yet it's still important to do so. Discuss available therapy options. If you aren't an oncologist or training to be one, you may have difficulty. If you're the patient's primary care physician, it's prudent to become familiar with the therapy options discussed by the oncologist.

WATCH OUT FOR...

Telling the family, not the patient

Beware the family who talks to you away from the patient with phrases like, "Come on, Doc, you can tell me," "What are the chances? I saw on the Internet that 60% of the patients don't survive past 18 months," and "Be honest, Doc." Speak to the family as you have with the patient and don't say things to the family that you haven't said to the patient.

Prevention and Preparation

By now, you might be thinking, "What about full disclosure? What about letting the patient prepare for death? What if the patient wants to discuss the possibility of dying or his or her concerns about dying? What about the survival statistics?" These are all good questions that you should be asking. A patient can benefit from speaking openly of impending death. Even so, your next question should be, "Will you destroy the patient's hope by speaking of the possibility that the therapy may not succeed?" In "Hope for the Best and Prepare for the Worst" from the March 4, 2003, issue of the *Annals of Internal Medicine,* Drs. Back, Arnold, and Quill offer guidelines to help you prepare for this situation. They make several recommendations, including:

- Give equal time to hoping and preparing.
- Align patient and physician hopes.
- Encourage but don't impose the dual agenda of hoping and preparing.
- Support the evolution of hope and preparation over time.
- Respect hopes and fears and respond to emotions.

What if . . . A patient or family member asks you tough questions that you aren't sure how to answer?

Although this situation is more likely to happen to you as a student or junior resident, it happens to practicing physicians more often than they would like to admit. As a student, the difficulty is commonly created by your stage of learning. For example, you may get a question about a medication the patient is taking that you aren't familiar with or a question about what is involved with an upcoming procedure the patient will be undergoing. As a practicing physician, the question may be in a subject area that is outside your area of expertise or may be a question the person learned from watching television dramas, such as "Doctor, how long do I have to live?" A major part of the difficulty in these situations is made worse by the expectation that the physician should know everything.

What To Do

There are four basic steps for dealing effectively with this situation:

- Listen carefully to the patient's question. We're not kidding! Our strong desire to meet a patient's expectations commonly makes us jump to premature conclusions and answer a question the patient didn't even ask.

- Ask clarifying questions to help you understand what the patient is asking or understand what the patient really wants to know, even if the question is vague or unfocused. Asking clarifying questions also gives you some time to think about your answer.
- Acknowledge areas of uncertainty and be honest about what you don't know. Make your best effort to answer the question, while being careful to avoid giving incorrect information.
- Finally, acknowledge and follow up on unanswered questions.

Regarding such questions as "How long do I have to live?" it's best never to try to predict the future. You'll likely be wrong and may not help the patient work toward a longer survival. At the same time, though, try to give the patient some idea of what to expect. More specifically, never reply with a prediction of how many days, months, or years the patient will survive. However, it's reasonable to discuss next steps regarding further diagnosis and treatment, difficulties that the patient may encounter along the way, and general survival trends based on research data.

 WARNING!!! It's important to remind the patient that, although research data describes population trends that have been studied, each patient is an individual whose outcome isn't restricted to the results of a particular study. (See the *What if* on page 157.)

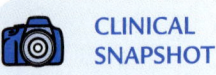 **CLINICAL SNAPSHOT**

Admit you're human

Perhaps you're a student who has just begun an elective rotation on the cardiology service and you're doing a history and physical on an admission. The patient happens to have an implantable cardioverter defibrillator and she asks you, "How often do I have to come to the hospital to have these batteries changed?" Options for a reply include, "I'm not sure but I'll check and get back to you," or "That may vary depending on the manufacturer, so I'll review your records, check with your primary cardiologist, and get back to you."

A similar scenario could happen if you're a resident, fellow, or practicing physician in a specialty other than cardiology and you're seeing this same cardiology patient in consultation. Your reply to the patient could be the same as previously described. You may also feel compelled to add that cardiology isn't your specialty, but that you'll make sure the patient's question gets answered.

WARNING!!! Don't fall into the trap of being defensive or worse yet, being offensive. "I really don't know your case that well," "I'm just a student," or "I don't have time today" are examples of being defensive. Chiding the patient for asking the question ("Weren't you listening to me when I told you the risks?") is offensive, as is blaming someone else ("I'm just covering for your doctor. He should have told you that.").

Prevention and Preparation

The best way to prepare for this *What if* scenario is to pause for a moment before seeing the patient. Think about the diagnosis, the prognosis, and what you'll say. Think about questions that you may be asked and possible answers you would provide. Such preparation enhances your effectiveness in helping this patient and helps you avoid falling into the "defensiveness-trap" described in the preceding warning.

What if . . .

You think a patient is faking?

This *What if* scenario isn't as unusual as you may think. Probably the most common situation of this kind is a patient who's exaggerating or lying about symptoms in order to gain time off from work or school or establish grounds for a worker's compensation or liability claim (sometimes referred to as *malingering*). On rare occasions, you'll encounter a patient who's suffering from a psychological disorder called *Munchausen syndrome,* which involves creating a factitious disease picture purely to become a patient. It's important to separate out patients who are knowingly misleading you from patients who are unaware that they're falsely describing symptoms. Those unaware patients are suffering from a conversion disorder and truly believe their reported symptoms, which can commonly be as severe as blindness, paralysis, or deafness with no actual organic deficit.

WARNING!!! Patients with apparent conversion disorder need psychiatric evaluation and treatment. Also be on the lookout for patients who may be deceitful because of a fear of what action will result, such as admission to the hospital, venipuncture, or other invasive procedure. Take care to address the patient's concerns and provide ample opportunity for the patient to ask questions. Also, consider providing more information about possible consequences of not treating the problem.

Unfortunately, some patients lie by fabricating or exaggerating signs and symptoms. You should suspect this scenario if a patient's history is vague or inconsistent, the complaints aren't consistent with physical findings (for example, stocking- or glovelike distribution of a complaint of numbness or sensory loss that doesn't correspond to anatomical dermatomes) or the disability is out of proportion to the problem (for example, a headache causing someone to be out of work for a year).

What To Do

Conduct a particularly careful examination and history of the complaint, using repetition as a tool. Ask the same questions multiple times in different ways. Inconsistent responses indicate misrepresentation. Examine the same body part in several ways, again looking for inconsistencies. Observe the patient's behavior carefully for inappropriateness (for example, "Oh yeah, doc, it's killing me," said with an air of nonchalance or a smile). There are many physical examination maneuvers you can use to determine if a patient is faking. Here, we'll cover a few of the most effective.

Too Weak to Walk

> ### MUNCHAUSEN SYNDROME
>
> Munchausen syndrome is named for Baron von Munchausen, an officer in the German military who was widely known for his grossly embellished stories about himself and his experiences. Patients with this problem repeatedly go to hospitals with symptoms severe enough to merit admission and work-up. Common presenting complaints are chest pain, abdominal pain, or fever that eventually becomes a fever of unknown origin (FUO). New symptoms are reported after the initial work-up is negative. Such a patient usually has a past history of multiple hospitalizations at different hospitals and commonly has several surgical scars from exploratory laparotomies. This syndrome is a complex mental illness that requires psychiatric evaluation and treatment. Another manifestation of the syndrome is called *Munchausen by proxy,* in which a parent repeatedly creates factitious or even real illness in a child.

A patient complaining of severe weakness or paralysis of an extremity should have abnormal deep tendon reflexes (hypoactive or hyperactive). If the weakness is prolonged there should be muscle atrophy, so measure the circumference of the affected limb and compare it to the opposite side. If the patient is complaining of a painful body part, take the patient's pulse before and after performing the maneuver that induces or worsens the pain. You should detect an increase in the pulse rate with valid pain (sometimes called *Mannkopf's sign*).

Numb or Dumb?

A commonly faked complaint is numbness or total loss of sensation on one side of the body, commonly the entire half of the body. Use the tuning fork vibratory sensation test on a bony prominence. With true paresthesia, anesthesia, or paralysis, vibratory sensation is usually intact. You can also use the tuning fork at the midline of the sternum to test the patient complaining of total anesthesia on one side of the body. Place the vibrating tuning fork on the midline but lean the distal end far to the left saying, "Can you feel this vibrating on this side?" Then test a metacarpal and then go back to the midline with the tuning fork leaning far to the right saying, "Can you feel it on this side?" If he says he can't feel it on one side, you know he's faking because you tested the same location. Another maneuver in the patient complaining of this "hemi-anesthesia" is to use light touch. Ask the patient to close his eyes and tell him, "Say 'yes' if I touch you and 'no' if I don't." A patient who truly has anesthesia in a location shouldn't say anything when you perform a light touch maneuver with a cotton swab in the affected area. Lastly, in the patient complaining of total paralysis of one leg, try Hoover's sign. With the patient in the recumbent position, stand at the foot of the bed, place your hands under the heel of each of the patient's feet and ask the patient to raise the affected leg keeping the knee extended. If the leg is truly paralyzed, your hand under the opposite heel will feel the downward pressure of the good leg while the patient is trying to lift the affected leg.

Weak Back About a Week Back

Another common scenario involves a complaint of severe back pain, typically on one side, right or left. With the patient in the recumbent position and keeping the knee extended, slowly lift the leg on the opposite side from the pain. You should be able to gain about 75° to 90° of flexion of the hip joint without producing back pain. Now try the leg on the affected side and note how many degrees of flexion of the hip joint you attain before the patient complains of back pain. The degree of flexion attained should be far less on the affected side and, if raising the leg doesn't produce back pain, either the pain isn't real or you're dealing with pain that's caused by something other than vertebral disc disease (such as renal colic). (Ruling out renal colic is fairly simple as patients who are suffering from it have a terrible time sitting still or laying down and will usually pace the room.) Next, examine another part of the body, then ask the patient to sit up and dangle his legs over the side of the examining surface. Repeat the straight-leg raising maneuver on both sides by grasping the patient's heel with one hand and holding down the ipsilateral knee joint with your other hand. This maneuver on the affected side should induce a pain response similar to the patient's response in the recumbent position. If no pain is elicited, the patient is likely faking.

No Free Passes Here

If you're confident that the patient is faking, have an honest conversation with him about your findings and how they don't make clinical sense. Giving the patient this information won't be well received, but it's a much better route to take than pretending the complaint is real. Typically, the patient will act in some way to remove himself from the scenario, especially if you're unwilling to write a note excusing him from work or supporting his claim.

Prevention and Preparation

Although it's hard to control someone else's behavior, it isn't altogether impossible. Make it clear to your patient that your approach to diagnosis is careful, thorough, data-driven, and quite serious. The "Hi! I wanna be your friend (not your doctor)" approach is not only inappropriate, but sends a signal to any fake that you're any easy mark. When signs and symptoms don't make sense or the severity of the complaint is inconsistent with the emotional condition of the patient, send a signal to that patient. A raised eyebrow and a comment such as "That's odd," or "That's unusual," can let the patient know that you aren't as gullible as he might think. You may just head-off any ploy coming your way.

What if . . .

You're developing inappropriate feelings toward a patient such as anger or attachment?

As a physician, approaching each patient objectively is essential to an accurate diagnosis and a rational therapeutic approach. However, physicians are only human and can have emotional reactions to patients (also humans). These reactions could be based simply (and wrongly) on a patient's country of origin, religion, race, or sexual preference, or perhaps the patient's hygiene leaves a lot to be desired. Objectivity is essential, however, and prejudice and discrimination are absolutely forbidden. Fortunately, these types of feelings rarely play a role in the patient-physician relationship. More common feelings include frustration and anger or, over a longer period, attachment.

What To Do

Always be self-aware and identify your feelings toward a patient. This process is usually easy if you remain clinically focused. Typical feelings for a patient include a combination of concern for his health, a desire to play a role in efficiently diagnosing and treating his problem, and a desire to provide information and reassurance to put him at ease.

Not So Easy

However, if you begin to realize that you're feeling frustrated or even angry with the patient, stop to reflect. What actions or inactions by the patient have been frustrating or anger provoking? Has he failed to comply with a medication regimen? Noncompliance should be addressed by gaining a better understanding of the reasons for the noncompliance. Does the patient understand the purpose of the medicine? Have you given him an understanding of how the medication or therapy works and why timing and regular doses are important? Is the patient having trouble affording the medication? Perhaps there is a less expensive alternative or some additional resources in the community that can help.

Is the patient frequently late or doesn't come to appointments? Discuss this issue with the patient and attempt to learn if there are some special circumstances that are causing the problem, such as transportation problems, work commitments, or dependent care responsibilities. If none of these obstacles are causing the problem, it's important to state clearly your expectations of the patient regarding timeliness and advanced notice for a cancellation. Psychiatrists usually take an approach referred to as the "50-minute hour," but this approach is harder to apply if you're rarely on time yourself. If you're always late, you have little grounds for expecting your patients to be on time. In fact, your lateness may actually be provoking some of the patient's lateness or missed appointments. Make your best effort to be on time and your patients will be more likely to do the same.

⊕ WATCH OUT FOR...

Rooting-for-the-patient trap

Don't fall for the "rooting-for-the-patient" trap. As a physician takes care of patients over a number of years, it isn't unusual to develop fondness for a few. This attachment is beyond compassion, which is appropriate. It can be an almost parental feeling of protection and hope that the patient doesn't develop a life-threatening disease. The trap lies in the potential to ignore symptoms or not order diagnostics because of an unconscious wish that the patient won't have a serious problem. A form of psychological denial can develop. A related phenomenon is a gradual change in the nature of the patient appointment. During each visit, more time is spent on discussions of family, vacations, and work and less time is spent on the history, signs and symptoms, and examination. Being aware of the potential for this trap is the main defense against falling into it.

Psychiatrists commonly follow a routine for office appointments that consists of a 50-minute hour. If the patient's appointment is for 1:00 p.m., then the patient has the time slot from 1:00 p.m. to 1:50 p.m. If the patient arrives, for example, at 1:35 p.m., the time slot from 1:35 p.m. to 1:50 p.m. is available to them. These strict rules for routine office visits are made clear to the patient during their first appointment and are adhered to with rare exception. (The 10 minutes from 1:50 p.m. to 2:00 p.m. are reserved for completing the medical record.)

Mirror, Mirror

If the cause for your unpleasant feelings isn't as simple as lateness or noncompliance or there seems to be no obvious cause, reflect again. It may be that you're mirroring the patient's feelings. The patient may be frustrated or angry with you. Look more closely. Is the patient harboring unpleasant feelings and not expressing them? Ask some leading questions, such as "You appear to be upset or concerned by our discussion or what I've said. Can you talk with me about that?" or "This discussion could easily cause difficult feelings for you. Can you tell me how you're feeling about what is happening?" Try to identify the patient's feelings and then help him express them and resolve them.

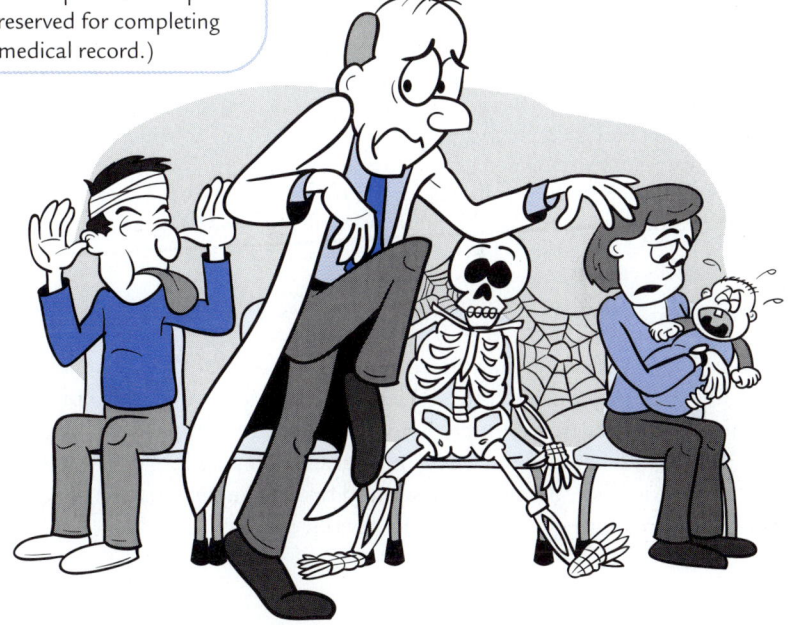

You're developing inappropriate feelings toward a patient such as anger or attachment? **169**

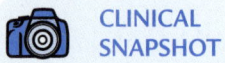

**CLINICAL
SNAPSHOT**

Exercise in frustration

Perhaps the most difficult type of situation is the patient who frustrates you because his noncompliance or other frustrating behavior is something he doesn't seem to see. He commonly has excuses for his behavior, which he believes are valid but test your patience. Here's how an exchange with such a patient might go:

Patient: "I missed my appointment because you always say I should be on time and I knew I was going to be late."
Doctor: "Why didn't you call to cancel the appointment?"
Patient: "I didn't want to bother you with a phone call."
Doctor: "Never hesitate to call."
A few weeks later
Doctor: "My answering service said you called. What's wrong?"
Patient: "I have to cancel my appointment."
Doctor: "Why is this an emergency?"
Patient: "It isn't. I never told the answering service that it was an emergency just that I really needed to speak with you."

If reading this paragraph is making you frustrated, that is the point! This illustrates interactions with what psychiatrists commonly called *passive-aggressive* personality disorder. Passive-aggressive people have a strong aversion to accepting responsibility without openly stating so. As with most personality disorders, these people are usually unaware and unwilling to be aware of their difficulties. They accept little responsibility for their behavior and commonly blame others for all of their problems. There are no tried-and-true approaches to therapy for this type of person. You should remain objective and use methods such as "the 50-minute hour" to avoid being manipulated.

Prevention and Preparation

Knowing yourself is a great step toward prevention of this *What if* scenario. Knowing your own shortfalls and what frustrates you or tends to provoke an emotional response from you helps you to avoid those traps. Be alert to behaviors that could bring out the worst in a patient. Finally, active listening, being clear in your discussions with patients, and taking the time to answer questions will pay off and are a good investment of your time.

Notes

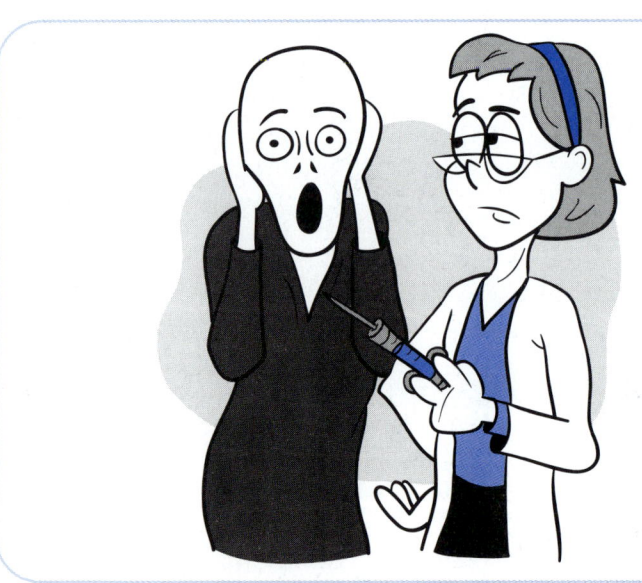

What if . . .

A patient is highly fearful of needles?

It isn't unusual for a patient to fear the needles used for phlebotomy, IV line insertions, subcutaneous or intramuscular (IM) injections, needle aspirations, and even those needles used to inject something to eliminate pain (local anesthetics). The origins of the fear may be multiple and range from a previous bad experience to being threatened with getting a shot for bad behavior as a child.

What To Do

If the patient alerts you to his fear or shows you signs that he may have a fear of needles, take the time to discuss the fear to see if there is an obvious cause. After listening carefully and asking appropriate questions to clarify, explain to the patient that you've learned the most comfortable way to give injections, draw blood, or perform needle aspirations.

 WARNING!!! The patient who says, "Oh, needles make me faint!" should be taken seriously. It's best to have this patient lie in the recumbent position as soon as possible after he makes this statement and proceed with your calming, pain-free approach.

Three Keys (or Gems) for Subcutaneous and IMs

There are three key secrets to performing subcutaneous and IM injections as painlessly as possible:

1. Warm no harm.
2. Touch; don't stab.
3. Slow as you go; fast gets gasps.

Warm and Cozy

Whenever possible, warm the solution or suspension you're injecting. Cold injections are far more painful, which is why dentists actually have special warmers for their local anesthetics. At the bedside, the simplest way to warm the vial is to hold it in your clenched hand while you're talking with the patient. Although the vial won't get to body temperature, it will be much warmer than when you picked it up.

Soft Touch

Far too many health-care providers misguidedly think that the quicker you get an injection over with, the easier it is on the patient. So, many simply stab the needle into the patient like a dart—sometimes even holding the syringe as though it were a dart. Instead, explain to the patient that you're going to gently lay the needle against his skin, so he can feel its touch instead of its bite. Then gently lay the needle (attached to the syringe) onto the skin at an oblique angle with the bevel edge facing away from the skin and not allowing the point of the needle to pierce the skin initially. Pause, then slowly introduce the needle through the skin to the appropriate depth (subcutaneous or IM). If you can,

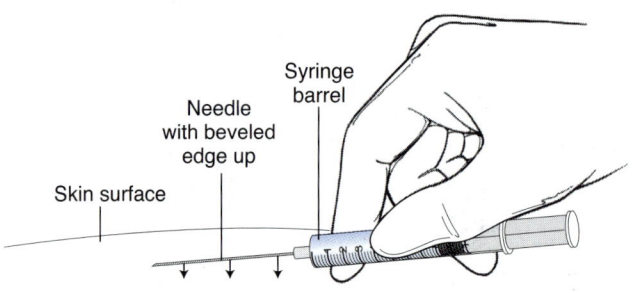

Syringe
barrel

Needle
with beveled
edge up

Skin surface

Initially, downward
movement and pressure
in the direction of these arrows

Pain-reducing injection method.

simultaneously with the insertion, use your other hand to touch the patient in another location on the arm. This maneuver attempts to use the "gate theory" of neurosensory transmission to block the painful sensation.

Slow and Steady

Aspirate briefly to make sure you aren't in a blood vessel. Then slowly—and—we mean *slowly*—inject the material. The more slowly you go, the better and less painful the injection will be. Stabbing and rapidly injecting is certainly easier on the provider but much more painful for the patient. Don't do it.

Phlebotomy or Needle Aspirations

Use the same "touch; don't stab" technique when introducing needles through a patient's skin for other procedures such as phlebotomy or needle aspirations. After you withdraw a phlebotomy needle, it's important to apply pressure to the puncture site with a sterile gauze pad.

 WARNING!!! Don't fall into the trap of applying the pressure before you withdraw the needle. If you apply the pressure while the needle is still in the vein, it will be more painful for the patient and may puncture the posterior wall of the vein.

Prevention and Preparation

Think through and find ways to practice the steps previously outlined. Keep in mind that dismissing needle punctures as a trivial, transiently painful moment for your patient is a mistake. The "grab, stab, and push" method is what caused your patient to fear needle punctures in the first place. If you use these pain-free techniques with young patients, they're less likely to develop fear of needles as adults. Moreover, approaching needle punctures responsibly can change the feelings of adults who've already had bad experiences and can enhance their ability to feel confident in their physician.

What if . . .

A patient threatens your life?

"I'm gonna kill you!" is a *What if* that occurs most commonly in the Emergency Department, but can also happen at the bedside, in the office, or even on the phone. Though there is a spectrum of such behavior, all violent and potentially violent patients should be taken quite seriously. Luckily, most violent patients usually issue what constitutes a "verbal warning."

What To Do

If the patient overtly threatens harm to you, leave the room as quickly as possible and get help from your security services or the police. Don't turn your back on the patient while you exit. If the patient attempts to leave, let him leave and don't get in between the patient and the exit. Don't attempt to determine if the patient has a weapon. Presume that he does have a weapon and get help. As quickly as possible, let others working in the area know that the patient is violent.

If the threat is less overt than *"I'm gonna kill you,"* don't be tempted to dismiss or ignore the threat. Bravery in this instance equals stupidity. Less overt threats, such as "I'm getting really angry," or "Don't push me, Doc," should be taken very seriously. Excuse yourself from the area, politely saying something like, "Excuse me for a moment, I'll be right back," and then return with help from security. Use your judgment. If you're uncomfortable, bring the security officer into the room with you. Explain your concern to the patient—for example, "I want to help you, but your anger causes me to seek assistance in protecting myself. That way I can focus on your medical problems." If you're less concerned, it may be satisfactory to simply post a security officer outside the exam room door. Keeping a reasonable distance from the patient (about 3 feet), begin the interview by asking the patient what is troubling him. If the patient seems just agitated or annoyed, it's reasonable to proceed cautiously with the interview without a security officer present. Again, keep your distance physically and remain alert to any sign of escalation in the patient's behavior.

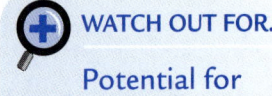

WATCH OUT FOR...

Potential for violence

Potentially violent patients are more likely to inflict violence on their children, spouse, friends, an elderly parent, or even themselves. There are multiple screening interviews that are used to identify patients or circumstances that have the potential for such violence. For more information, check out the entry on pediatric abuse on page 201.

Prevention and Preparation

Being alert to patients and situations that have the potential for violent behavior is the key to prevention. High alert circumstances include patients with drug or alcohol intoxication or withdrawal, paranoid schizophrenia, a history of violent behavior, hypoglycemia, or severe agitation or those that appear to be having trouble controlling themselves. Approach these patients with respect and concern. Don't ignore them or their behavior. Don't be confrontational physically or verbally. Try to get them to talk about why they're upset. Try to address their concerns and get them the help that they need.

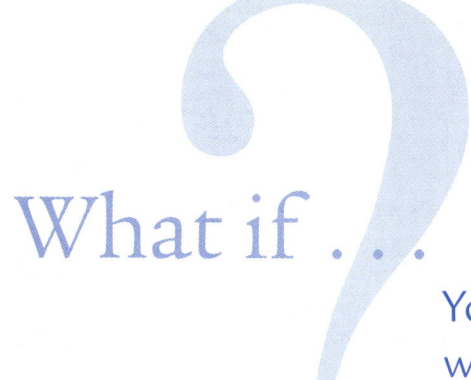

What if . . .

Your patient is upset with the care you're providing?

Occasionally, a patient or family is unhappy with the care you're providing and can become confrontational and, commonly, threaten a lawsuit. Your reflexive response may include embarrassment, defensiveness, regret, and fear. The fear may be for your own safety or, more likely, fear of a malpractice suit or a complaint filed with the state licensing board. This kind of response usually makes matters worse and can lead to arguing with the patient, blaming someone else, or even blaming the patient. Although it's a normal, human reaction, this reflexive response never yields a good outcome to this awkward situation.

 WARNING!!! If you don't want to read this *What if,* you definitely should! If you think this topic is silly or a waste of time, it may be a sign that you have a greater need to read it than the average caregiver. Arrogance is a dangerous disease in a health-care professional.

What To Do

Immediately offer to discuss the patient's concerns and suggest moving the discussion to a private area. Resistance to a change of venue can be overcome by expressing your desire to give full attention to the patient's concerns while protecting his or her privacy. When you've moved the discussion, ask the patient to express his concerns. Be an attentive, active listener. Take notes on specific concerns. Repeat the concerns you identify back to the patient to show that you're listening and understand. Ask clarifying questions. Most patient complaints are caused by lack of communication or misunderstanding.

When you've identified specific concerns, discuss them openly. Clear up misunderstandings. Be open and honest about what you can do to address concerns and what you aren't able to do. If there are some specific ways the patient can help solve the problem, point them out. For example, ask the patient to try hard to tell you when he or she doesn't understand what you're saying. Try to come to an agreement on what should be done to solve the problem and prevent future problems. Doing so establishes an informal contract between you and the patient, which gives you a chance to set reasonable expectations. For example, such expectations may refer to the patient's behavior or compliance with a medication regimen or expectations that you'll explain things more clearly.

Prevention and Preparation

According to Hickson's study published in the June 12, 2002, issue of *JAMA,* the risk of a mal-

THINGS TO REMEMBER

Do's and Don'ts of facing criticism

This checklist will help you take advantage of opportunities and avoid pitfalls when facing patient criticism.

Do's

- Listen carefully to a patient's questions.
- Return a patient's phone calls.
- Establish expectations for you and the patient.
- Time invested in discussion is worth its weight in gold!

Don'ts

- Don't be defensive.
- Don't blame the patient or family.
- Don't lose your temper.
- Don't refuse to discuss the problem.
- Don't be condescending. Education and experience don't give you the right to be arrogant, insulting, or accusatory.
- Don't walk away or cut the discussion short due to your time constraints.

practice suit appears, among other factors, "to be related to patients' dissatisfaction with their physician's ability to establish rapport, provide access, administer care and treatment consistent with expectations, and communicate effectively." What's more, the study found that the number of unsolicited patient complaints a physician receives is associated with a higher number of lawsuits, risk-management file openings, and file openings with expenditures. Instead of becoming overly defensive, view patient complaints as an incredible opportunity to improve care and reduce your chances of a lawsuit. Making this extra effort to communicate openly and often with patients and their families pays off and enhances your relationship with the patient.

ACME MEDICAL SCHOOL
DR. NO
DR. NO
THERE'S A MR. BOND HERE TO SEE YOU...
UH, OH...
DR. NO
DR. NO
DR. NO

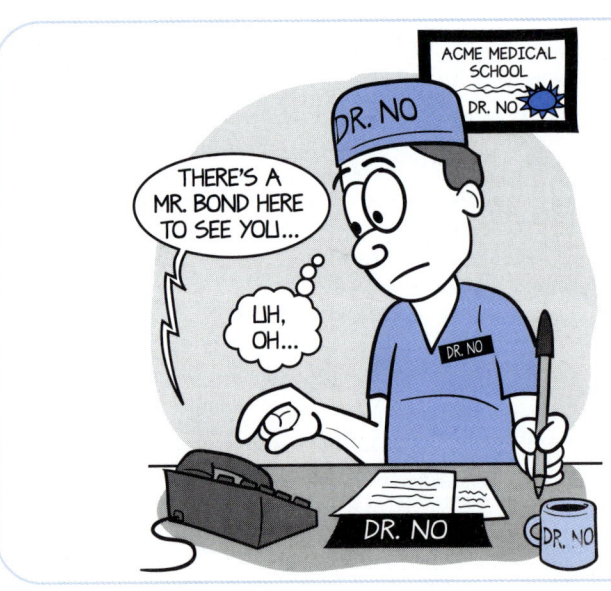

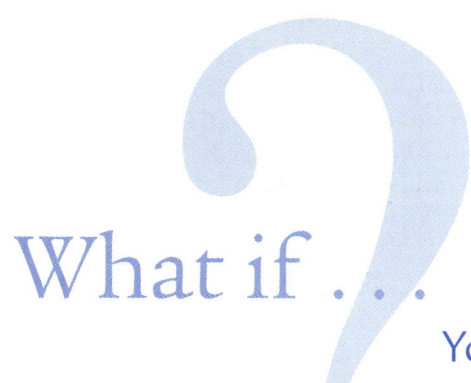

What if . . .

You have to say "no" to a patient's request?

At first blush, the answer to this question seems too simple to be a *What if* scenario. Why not *just say "no"*? However, as you provide care to more patients, you'll encounter some challenging situations and will be more likely to fall into a trap or two. Examples of this scenario include patients seeking narcotic pain medications, patients wanting to take prescription medications they've seen in television advertising or on the Internet, and patients who want you to write notes excusing them from work.

What To Do

The previous examples are a good way to consider approaches to this *What if.*

Patient Seeking Narcotics

The patient who is new to you and is seeking "something strong" for pain relief usually has back pain, severe headache, or sometimes is passing a kidney stone. You'll commonly encounter these types of patients in the emergency department of a hospital or at an urgent care walk-in center. In addition, a patient with one of these complaints may also be seen by a doctor who specializes in the problem, such as an orthopedist, urologist, neurologist, neurosurgeon, or even an internist or family practitioner. This *What if* can't cover a thorough evaluation of these complaints; however, we can discuss a few tips. In each of these situations, use all of your observation skills to assess the validity and extent of the patient's problem. Beware of the patient who doesn't seem to be suffering from as much pain as he claims. In addition to having at least microscopic hematuria, a patient who is passing a kidney stone can't sit or lie still for long and gets up frequently to pace the floor. Patients with severe headache, such as a migraine, will usually have photophobia, nausea or vomiting, and commonly visual disturbances. If a patient tells you she rarely has headaches and this one is the absolute worst she has had in her life, you should seriously consider subarachnoid or cerebral hemorrhage.

The clincher is when you tell the patient that you're going to write a prescription for a nonsteroidal anti-inflammatory agent and the patient replies, "Gee, doc, the only one that works for me is the yellow pill," (usually Percodan or Percocet), or "My doctor back home says I need something strong like that Oxy one," (OxyContin). Then is the time to just say no, and explain that you *never* write prescriptions for those medications. (See the entry on page 163 for more information on patients who may be faking.)

WARNING!!! The postoperative patient who's asking for another refill on narcotic pain medication may be having continued serious pain or may be in danger of addiction or severe habituation. Most surgical patients can easily move from a narcotic pain medication to acetaminophen or ibuprofen within a few days of surgery. So, if a postoperative patient calls and pushes for more narcotics, it's best to ask him to come in to be seen. He may be in the early stages of a wound infection or may be developing a slow growing hematoma or other postoperative complication.

Patient Seeking Drugs Seen on TV or the Internet

The amount of direct-to-consumer advertising of prescription drugs has grown immensely in

WATCH OUT FOR...

The easy way out

Don't fall into the trap of taking the easy way out as a time-saver. Yes, saying "no" does take more time and may not be as pleasant; nevertheless, it's worth the time invested. Don't be afraid to lose the patient to another physician. Any patient who abandons you after you've taken the time to evaluate his condition and explain your decision isn't a good match for your practice. There are many other patients who are!

the past few years. Many of these ads are vague, such as for "social anxiety dis-order," but the images presented are so pleasant, the patient wonders if she should be taking the drug. The patient will commonly arrive with a print out from the Internet that she'll use to argue the case. At least the Internet material gives you enough information to understand the proper indications for the drug. From there, you should use your diagnostic skills to determine if this drug is appropriate for your patient. Keep in mind that the patient may be try-ing to tell you that her current medication isn't working, so make sure you ex-plore that possibility! Explain your answer to the patient in clear terms that show her you aren't dismissing the suggestion without considering it carefully.

Patient Seeking Excuse From Work

It's far too easy to go along with a patient who wishes to be excused from work. You should evaluate the clinical situation objectively and make a determina-tion about whether the patient is really ill enough to stop working. If your con-clusion is yes, formulate a plan for reevaluating the patient's return-to-work capability in an appropriate period of time. Keep in mind the difficulties caused by someone in your office staying out of work unnecessarily. It's perfectly rea-sonable to decline this request and explain why it isn't appropriate to be out of work for the particular illness or injury.

Prevention and Preparation

Make every effort to establish good rapport with the patient when you first en-counter him. It makes it easier if you have to say "no" to a request. Be alert to signs that the request is coming and use soft, preemptive phrases before the pa-tient makes the request, such as "Luckily, this type of injury won't cause you to miss work," or, "This type of pain responds well to ibuprofen."

What if . . .

A patient refuses treatment?

A patient refusing treatment is a common occurrence. A patient may be reluctant to have surgery, chemotherapy, or radiation therapy for cancer. She may also decide to leave the hospital inpatient service or emergency department *against medical advice.* The reason a patient refuses treatment is usually based on a lack of appropriate information, which can lead to fear of the treatment or procedure. The refusal may also result from a lack of confidence in the physician. How a physician reacts to and approaches a patient's refusal is a major factor in solving this problem.

What To Do

Patience and understanding are first and foremost in approaching a patient who has refused treatment. Don't react abruptly, judgmentally, or with condescension. Instead, gently ask the patient why she refused treatment. Be prepared for a reply that may not get to the root of the problem. Follow up by asking the patient what she feels will happen if she agrees to go forward with the treatment or procedure. You may need to describe what you think she might be feeling to get her to open up and discuss her feelings. Acknowledge her concerns and how well you understand why she's feeling that way. If the patient describes her concerns well, you can attempt to fill any gaps in understanding that she might have. Also, make sure you're using lay-terms that are easily understood.

Happy Medium

Don't react with indignation, anger, frustration, or indifference. Over the past several decades, there has been an evolution in the nature of the doctor-patient relationship. The old, paternalistic, "doctor-knows-best" approach has given way to informed and active participation by the patient in key care and treatment decisions. Even so, don't go to the opposite extreme by abdicating responsibility for these decisions. You have a responsibility to provide good information to your patient to help her give an *informed* consent or *informed* refusal. In addition, the patient may ask for your opinion about what she should do. Don't avoid answering or offering your expert medical opinion. You have a responsibility to provide that as well.

When the conversation is flowing, allow the patient plenty of opportunity to ask additional questions. Be open and honest about potential complications or unpleasant side effects. Be clear about potential benefits but don't make any guarantees. There are no guarantees in medicine. Ask the patient to state in her own words what she thinks you're saying. Doing so will help you determine if the patient understands what you're discussing.

Increase the Odds

You may need to give the patient some time to think through your discussion of the information. Return at a later point, depending on the urgency of the clinical situation, to answer additional questions and ask again for her permission to go forward. If you've followed these guidelines, you'll have carried out

INFORMED CONSENT AND ADVANCE DIRECTIVES

If the patient is incapacitated enough to seriously impair comprehension of the discussion and make it unlikely that you'll obtain a truly informed consent, you'll need to speak with the patient's family. Before you do so, though, be sure to check to see if the patient has established an advance directive to address such a situation.

An advance directive usually delineates what extreme measures a patient would be willing to or would like to have done or, sometimes, what the patient isn't willing to have done. The laws of the state in which the patient is located govern the use of a patient's advance directives. Sometimes the advance directive will designate a surrogate decision-maker for the "incompetent patient." In some states, that person is called the *health-care proxy.* In other states, that person is given a *health-care power of attorney.* If an incompetent patient has no next-of-kin or designated health-care proxy or power of attorney, a *guardianship* is determined by a court upon petition from a hospital or other health-care facility.

Familiarize yourself with the resources at your facility, such as the risk management department, that can assist you with these legal issues. And remember, although it's tempting to consult with the family of an incompetent patient, be sure to check for advance directives before approaching the family.

a proper *informed consent* and will have the best chance of having the patient agree to the treatment or procedure.

Prevention and Preparation

The best method for preventing this difficult *What if* is to take the time to fully acquaint yourself with the patient and give the patient information to allow her to get acquainted with you. Explain as much as possible about diagnosis and treatment options, answer her questions, and be alert to the patient's level of anxiety. As a way to test the patient's understanding and anxieties, ask the patient to repeat back key pieces of information you have conveyed. If she's unable to do it well, you'll need to revisit the issue and strive to help the patient better understand the proposed treatment. Remember, knowledge is power; so give your patient the knowledge she needs to make the right decision.

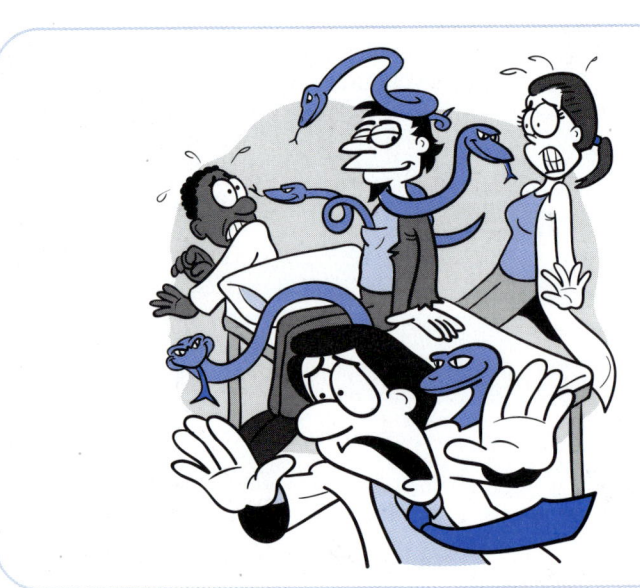

What if . . .

A patient is a herpetophile and brings a pet snake into the exam room?

SNAKE MISTAKES

The rattlesnake, cottonmouth, and copperhead are the venomous or poisonous snakes found in North America. These snakes have a catlike pupil (vertical slit) in their iris, whereas nonpoisonous snake pupils are round. It isn't uncommon for novice amateur herpetophiles to fail to realize that the rattlesnake they have "defanged" will regrow fangs and can even inject venom with the more posterior teeth. For more information on how to handle a venomous snakebite, see the *What if* on page 231.

If this seems like a somewhat outrageous *What if,* that's because it is! Nevertheless, this can and has happened. In certain parts of Tennessee, Kentucky, Virginia, West Virginia, North Carolina, Alabama, and Georgia, some religious groups practice snake or serpent handling. More common, though, are amateur herpetologists who keep snakes—usually poisonous snakes—as pets and typically want to show off their pets and their ability to handle them.

What To Do

Keep a prudent distance between you and the snake. Ask the patient what kind of snake it is. Compliment the patient on the unusual pet and the patient's ability to handle snakes. Then politely ask the patient to take the snake out of the building. If the patient has brought a cage or other "snake-carrying" device, ask the patient to place the snake into the cage before going through areas of the building where there are other people. Explain that other people are usually frightened by snakes and may take actions that could frighten or even harm the snake.

With good intentions, the patient will likely try to reassure you that the snake is perfectly harmless. He may even ask you to handle the snake in order to demonstrate the validity of his assertion of the benign nature of his pet. Don't do it! Though most snakes native to North America are nonvenomous and up to 25% of venomous snakebites are "dry," there is still a risk of tissue damage and secondary infection from a nonvenomous bite. Most snake bites happen on the hands and fingers of people who keep and handle snakes.

Prevention and Preparation

To find out more about snake handling and cultures that practice snake handling, check out *Serpent Handling Believers* by Thomas Burton (1993, Knoxville: University of Tennessee Press). For more information on dealing with snakebite victims, see the chapter on "Snakebite" in *Conn's Current Therapy* (2006, Philadelphia: W.B. Saunders Co.).

TAKING UP SERPENTS

George Went Hensley is often considered to be the originator (if only by himself) of religious serpent handling. In the early part of the 20th century in East Tennessee, Hensley is said to have been presented with a box full of rattlesnakes during a sermon on the book of the Bible, Mark 16. He immediately picked up several of the snakes and continued preaching unscathed. "And these signs shall follow them that believe: in my name they shall cast out devils; they shall speak with new tongues; they shall take up serpents and if they drink any deadly thing, it shall not hurt them . . . " Though snake handling is part of a complex religious belief of some Christian sects and should be taken seriously, please note that Mr. Hensley died in 1955—from a snake bite.

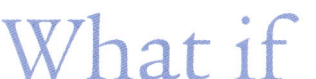

What if . . .

You have to give a family very bad news?

It's always difficult to convey bad news to a patient's family. Whether it's telling a patient's loved one that the patient has died or is gravely ill, or discussing a cancer diagnosis, there is no easy way. Although you usually won't encounter this situation as a student, the lack of training on this subject can make any clinician anxious.

What To Do

Properly conveying a patient's death to the patient's family or a loved-one is difficult; however, it's important to do so in a manner that helps the family begin the grieving process properly.

 WARNING!!! Be aware that you have your own personal feelings about and experiences with death or severe loss. Think about those feelings in advance to avoid getting lost in those feelings while trying to help a patient's family.

First, it's important to get the family into a private area or room. They should be seated and you should sit down to speak with them. Next, consider the circumstances. Is this the long-anticipated death of a cancer victim who has suffered for a period of time or is this a sudden, unexpected death? Families experiencing long-anticipated deaths have had time to begin the grieving process and are usually at a point where they can better accept the loss and acknowledge the patient's relief from suffering. Your approach should incorporate the most likely feelings associated with the circumstances.

In either instance, though, your first sentence should get right to the point. You might start out with "I'm sad to say that, despite all our efforts, Mr. Smith has passed away. He wasn't in any pain at the end." Depending on the circumstances, it's usually appropriate to speak of some of those efforts that were unsuccessful and also to convey that the patient's passing was peaceful and as painless as possible. It's likely that the next few sentences you speak won't really be heard. So, pause after a few sentences and be silent. If there are no questions or if someone moves quickly to a comment such as, "Well, thank you doctor," then ask them if they have any questions for you. Use your observation skills to assess how they're coping. Some may want to visit the patient one more time, especially if the death is unexpected. For long-anticipated deaths associated with suffering, it's usually comforting to the family to be reminded that the patient's suffering is over. Even in the case of a long-anticipated death, however, there is typically a tremendous amount of disbelief that the person is gone. In the intensity of the moment, don't forget to offer your sincerest condolences.

The grieving process can begin when the person is forewarned of the impending death. The anticipation of this loss and the thinking process leading up to the death are generally therapeutic. It's beneficial if the family can be present at the time of death and can help with final caring for the patient.

Be supportive as well as alert to factors that may predispose someone to having a very difficult grieving process. Psychosocial support and therapy may be indicated if the situation involves such factors as a history of depression, an

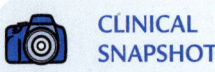

CLINICAL SNAPSHOT

No more secrets

Beware the family who says, "You mustn't tell him he has cancer!" Our first striking encounter with this scenario was when we accompanied a geriatric psychiatrist on a home-visit to a patient with cancer. The patient's wife and her sisters ushered us into the kitchen, and cheerfully offered us coffee and cookies. When we mentioned the subject of our patient's illness, his wife ignored us and her sister whispered, "Please speak softly. He doesn't know he has cancer. If he found out, it would kill him."

While we distracted the ladies with strange ER cases, the psychiatrist slipped into the living room where the patient was resting. The psychiatrist asked him, "How are you doing?" The man put his finger to his lips, pointed to the kitchen, and whispered, "Shhh, I'm dying but, whatever you do, don't tell them." The psychiatrist discussed with the patient the importance of telling his family and suggested that they probably already suspected it. Next, the psychiatrist spoke with the wife about the situation, and then brought the patient and wife together for an open, specific conversation.

unexpected death, a weak or lacking social support system, or the death of a child.

All Above-Board

Don't discuss a cancer diagnosis with a patient's family until you have thoroughly discussed it with the patient or the patient and the spouse together. There shouldn't be any behind-the-scenes discussion of information you haven't given the patient. In less common situations in which the patient doesn't have the capability to listen and discuss the diagnosis, you can discuss it with the family. For more information, follow the guidelines described in the *What if* on page 157.

Prevention and Preparation

As much as possible, try to anticipate the family's reaction to the circumstances of a death or difficult cancer diagnosis. The long-anticipated death of an elderly person who has had a full life is tolerated much more readily than the death of a child or young person. Try to prepare families in advance, even if it's only an hour in advance.

The "D" Word

You may have noticed the words *death* and *dying* used repeatedly in this *What if.* Yet, clinicians and support professionals commonly use substitute words, such as *loss, passed away, in time of need,* and *going away* or *gone.* Don't be afraid to use the terms *death* and *dying;* they help avoid confusion about what you're saying. In addition, if you struggle to find substitutes, your discomfort may make the patient or family uncomfortable, too. As humans we're about living and dying. Frank, compassionate communication of this universal truth with patients and their families will help them face this challenge together with dignity and understanding.

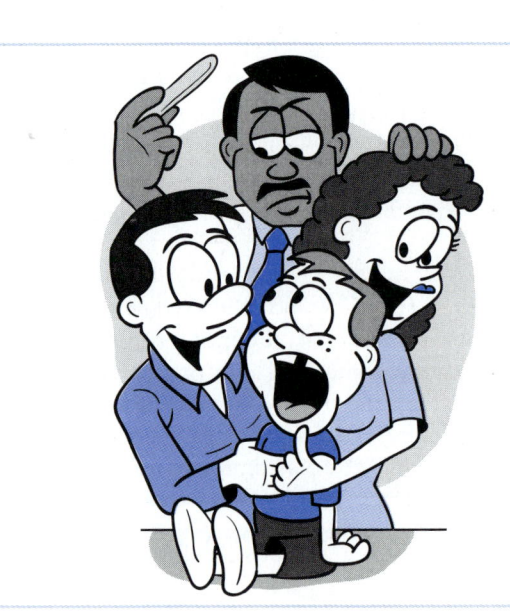

What if . . .

The presence of a young child's parents is getting in the way?

A child's parents can be the best resource when that child becomes your patient. Parents are usually your first choice for obtaining the history of the present illness and the child's past medical history. But parents can also be your biggest obstacle in the process of examining and treating a pediatric patient. For example, a child old enough to answer questions will do so, but commonly not in the presence of his parents. The mildly injured child (abrasion or small laceration) who's screaming will commonly be brave and relatively calm when the parents aren't present. In fact, it's observed and acknowledged by many parents that their child's behavior is more difficult when they're around.

Suffice it to say, the dynamic between child and parent is extremely complex and highly variable from family to family. The child who's a "finicky eater" eats well on a day-trip with an aunt and uncle. The child with typically bad behavior at home is usually just fine in school. An 8-year-old can't sleep without his parents but sleeps well alone during a visit with grandparents.

Today's parents are far more protective of their children than in past generations. The content of the media certainly indicates that this protectiveness is with good cause. Regardless, there are times in a clinical encounter when there is some benefit to interviewing a child or administering treatment without the

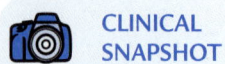

Laceration and doting parents

A very common clinical situation involves the toddler who has fallen at home and hit his chin on a coffee table or similar furniture. The result is almost invariably a linear, transverse laceration just under the child's chin. In a calm voice, speak with the child and parents about the event, clarifying the cause of the injury and establishing that there was no loss of consciousness after or seizurelike activity before or after the injury.

First, the parents
Next, walk the parents out of the exam room, leaving the child with your assistant, and explain to the parents that you'll need to use local anesthesia and then suture the laceration. Explain that this usually goes better with the parents not in the room. Also, explain that some evidence suggest that the presence of the parents during such a procedure can cause the child to resent the parents for allowing it to happen. Tell the parents you'll bring them back into the room to examine the sutured laceration before it's bandaged.

Then, the child
When dealing with the child, it's most important to use a technique that is as painless as possible to anesthetize and suture the wound. Also, speak to the child in a

presence of the parents. Some examples include circumstances in which you suspect child abuse (as in the *What if* on page 201.) or when you're trying to administer an injection or clean and dress an abrasion.

What To Do

Obviously, you'll spend time with the child and parents together, getting the chief complaint and history of the present illness and past medical history. Use this time as your opportunity to establish rapport with the parents and use your skills as a trained observer. The child who appears extremely frightened when the circumstances don't merit such fear or is screaming inappropriately may benefit from a brief interview without the parents or may calm down if the parents leave the room.

You must obtain permission from the parents to interview the child alone. Be clear up front that you will be accompanied by another trained health profes-

calming voice. Describe the sensations the child may feel just before the child may feel them. Use sterile drapes to protect the site, but also use the drapes to cover the child's eyes and keep the child from seeing such instruments as needles, scissors, and clamps.

Before injecting the local anesthetic, apply some of the anesthetic topically to the subcutaneous tissues by squirting the anesthetic onto the tissue or using a small amount to irrigate the wound. Tell the child there will be a feeling like cold water. Wait a minute or two to allow some topical anesthetic effect, then inject the anesthetic. Don't inject the anesthetic through the skin; rather, inject it into the subcutaneous tissue through the open wound. Remember to use the painless injecting technique described in the *What if* on page 174. Warm the anesthetic and inject it very slowly. Forewarn the child that there will be a slight burning sensation.

Allow time for the anesthetic to take effect. Take your time and slowly irrigate the wound with saline, again warning the child of the sensation of cold water. If the child reacts as you attempt to place the first suture, wait a few minutes or use some additional local anesthetic. However, don't exceed recommended dosages for the child's size (weight or body surface area).

Mission accomplished
When you have completed the repair, follow through and bring the parents in to examine the wound. Be sure to praise the child in front of the parents.

sional (such as a nurse, medical assistant, or clinical social services professional). Many times, the nurse or other professional can be helpful and reassuring to the parents. When requesting the parents' permission, explain the following:

- This is part of your routine in evaluating and treating pediatric patients.
- You'll be assisted by another trained health-care professional.
- You'll go over any findings with the parents.
- You'll discuss and obtain permission from the parents for any treatment or change in treatment from what you've already discussed.
- This approach is usually beneficial to the child and to the parent-child relationship.

 WARNING!!! You should consider a parent's refusal to allow you to be with the child without the parent as a warning sign of possible child abuse. You'll need the assistance of a social service professional if the parent refuses.

Prevention and Preparation

Upon first contact with the child's parents, reach out to establish a good relationship with them. Be friendly and engaging from the start. Give them tons of information. Answer all of their questions. Don't give them any of that "I'm the doctor, I know best" attitude. Don't give them the serious, stern, silent treatment nor behave as though they don't exist. These bad actions will only create a huge gap between you and the parents, a gap you'll have to try to cross eventually.

What if . . .

You think a pediatric patient is a victim of abuse?

Child abusers and abused children can be of any age, sex, race, appearance, profession, or socioeconomic class. So don't rule out abuse just because the child is the teenaged, designer-clothing-clad heir to the Chocolate candy empire. And certainly don't exclude abuse if the family appears to be upstanding citizens. They can turn into virtual Mr. or Mrs. Hydes at home or someone else (such as another family member, a nanny, a neighbor, a coach, or a teacher) is perpetrating the abuse.

Abuse can be physical (deliberately causing bodily harm), sexual (exposing or subjecting the child to any inappropriate sexual materials or situations), or emotional (such as blaming, humiliating, or ignoring the child to the point that it damages self-esteem). It can result from active attacks or neglect (failing to provide a reasonable level of care, such as adequate housing, clothing, supervision, food, emotional support, education, or hygiene).

What To Do

If you're a pediatrician and suspect child abuse, you're legally obligated to report your suspicions to your local community, clinic, or hospital child protective services. If you're a medical student or physician-in-training, relay your suspicions to your supervisor as soon as possible. Remember, you never know when abuse may lead to serious physical or emotional damage or even death. In some cases, you may be the child's only hope to end the abuse.

Keep in mind that you aren't responsible for confirming whether the abuse actually occurred, identifying the perpetrator, or determining when, how, or why it happened. Child protective services, child abuse specialists, and the police can handle these details. So resist any temptation to sleuth around for clues. When interviewing the child and parents (if they're in the room) and documenting your findings, be objective and don't render any opinions or judgments. For example, if you see a suspicious injury, just ask the child and family how it occurred and document what they say. Don't question their answers or criticize them. Don't tell the child's family that you suspect abuse—especially if you're a medical student or physician-in-training. Confronting the family requires expertise and experience that you likely don't have.

What's the risk in rendering premature judgments? First of all, no matter how bizarre the injury may seem or how "suspicious" you find the family, abuse may not have occurred, and you may be making false accusations, which, of course, isn't nice and may have significant legal ramifications. Second, even if abuse did occur, you may be accusing or implicating the wrong people. Third, if abuse did occur and the family members who are present perpetrated or condoned the abuse, they may leave with the child or "cover up" the evidence

DETECTING ABUSE

Abuse can be difficult to detect or confirm because there are no definitive signs or symptoms of abuse. Substance abuse, apathy, hostility, eating disorders, nightmares, bedwetting, antisocial behavior, problems in school, fear of adults, self-destructive or suicidal behavior, depression, and lack of self-esteem are potential clues that some type of abuse may have occurred. Physical injuries out of proportion to the explanation provided (for example, the child bumped his head on the cabinet and fractured his skull), injuries in the shape of an object (such as a cigar, belt, chain, or poker), bite marks, or repeated injuries raise suspicion of physical abuse. Children who display an inappropriate level of interest or lack of interest in sexuality, sexual information, and sexual acts may have been sexually abused. Also, be vigilant of children who act seductive or dress in a revealing manner. Neglected children may appear dirty, improperly clothed, hungry, or wild and uncontrollable.

before the proper services and authorities are notified.

If you suspect child abuse or neglect, call your local or state Child Protective Services (CPS) agency. If your city or state doesn't have a CPS agency, try the Childhelp USA National Child Abuse Hotline at 1-800-4-A-CHILD (1-800-422-4453).

In addition, the following organizations can provide extensive information and lists of other resources and organizations:

- National Clearinghouse on Child Abuse and Neglect Information, Children's Bureau, Administration for Children and Families Information
Address: 1250 Maryland Avenue, SW
Eighth Floor
Washington, DC 20024
Phone: 800-394-3366 OR 703-385-7565
E-mail: nccanch@caliber.com
Website:
http://nccanch.acf.hhs.gov/index.cfm
- The American Academy of Pediatrics
Address: 141 Northwest Point Boulevard
Elk Grove Village, IL 60007-1098
Phone: 847-434-4000
E-mail: kidsdocs@aap.org
Website: *http://www.aap.org*

Prevention and Preparation

Every hospital and clinic serving pediatric patients should have access to some type of Child Protective Services. Many pediatric hospitals will actually have a Child Abuse Team, consisting of pediatricians, nurses, psychiatrists, psychologists, and social workers specializing in these situations. Your facility's pediatrics department should know how to reach these services.

Learn how to remain calm and objective when dealing with emotionally charged situations. Getting angry at or voicing your opinions to the patient's family probably won't help and will potentially hurt the child. Consider shadowing your medical school or facility's child abuse specialists to get acclimated to the problem, so that you don't react emotionally the first time you encounter such a situation.

Get into the habit of asking all your pediatric patients about their general behavior, habits, interests, development, schoolwork, and social life. The answers may be the only initial clues of abuse. Remember, your role in these situations is to detect potential abuse, not to confirm, resolve, or campaign against the problem. Otherwise, instead of saving the child, you may be doing further damage to him or innocent family members.

OOPS...

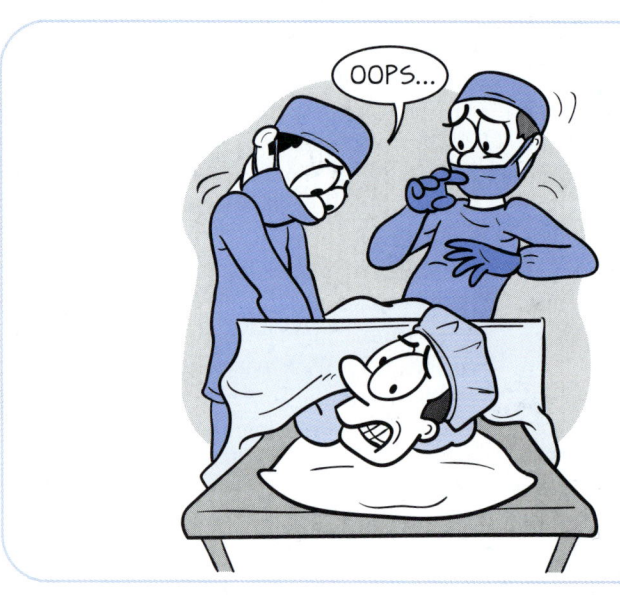

What if . . .

You make a mistake with a patient?

Although you hope it's a rare scenario, there are countless possibilities for making a mistake with a patient, such as ordering the wrong medication for a patient with a known allergy, performing surgery on the wrong extremity, leaving a sponge or instrument in an operative site, failing to order a chest x-ray after a particular procedure, such as placing a central line or tapping a pleural effusion. Specific clinical actions you should take if these mistakes are made are too numerous to address here; however, one of the key questions is universal: How do you approach the patient and family?

For too many years, the saying "Doctors bury their mistakes" was more truth than cynicism. Traditionally, doctors and hospitals have kept such medical errors under cover and haven't disclosed these errors to patients and their families. In the past, malpractice insurers were adamantly opposed to disclosure of any error and counseled and typically insisted that no such disclosures be made.

However, over the last 4 to 5 years, this scenario has changed tremendously. Research and experience are indicating that disclosures and apologies for medical errors can reduce the incidence of malpractice suits and the size of financial settlements. Surveys of patients have found an almost universal desire to know about mistakes that are made and nearly as strong an expectation of a sincere apology from the providers of the medical error. Even many malpractice insurers have become more receptive to—and even supportive of—appropriate disclosure and apologies.

What To Do

Don't panic. Stay calm. Make sure you take the appropriate clinical action to minimize consequences, including summoning help from other colleagues. When the clinical situation is under control (or, sometimes, simply ends), you're faced with the task of informing the patient and family (or deciding whether you should inform them). Should you disclose what happened? Should you apologize? Should you admit guilt or place blame? Here are some answers to these questions:

1. Ask for assistance from your institution's risk manager or a trusted colleague and review your facility's policies on disclosure.
2. Plan what will be said and by whom, who will be present, the appropriate private setting—all should be planned in advance.
3. Convey what is known at this time. Don't wait until your investigation is complete. Don't be defensive. Don't try to forecast the outcome of an investigation.
4. Sincerely apologize for the error that has occurred. Don't blame anyone or confess guilt until all facts are fully known. Be prepared for a spectrum of reactions from the patient or family, such as anger, disappointment, and gratitude.
5. Convey what steps will be taken and a method and point-person for follow-up conversation, conveying further information, and answering subsequent questions.
6. Be supportive and offer counseling, referral to another physician and, in most instances, assurance that the patient won't be billed for further care needed as a result of the error.

Prevention and Preparation

There are some basic measures you can take to try to prevent errors in your clinical practice. For example, make sure that you get an adequate amount of sleep each night and try to eat foods that won't adversely affect you or your ability to concentrate. What's more, take a moment before visiting each patient to ensure that you're alert and focused on that patient's condition.

The Massachusetts Coalition on the Prevention of Medical Errors has launched a project on accountability for patient safety. The goals of this project are to develop and implement a standard method of error reporting to patients as well as government and nongovernment agencies that require some type of error reporting. This project is a huge undertaking and a giant leap forward in disclosure practices. Check it out at *http://www.macoalition.org/initiatives.shtml.*

To prepare for the possibility of having to disclose an error, first become aware of your facility's policy regarding disclosure. In 2001, the Joint Commission for the Accreditation of Healthcare Organizations (JCAHO) issued a standard that requires disclosure of serious errors. Since then, the majority of hospitals have established policies on disclosure of medical errors to patients. In addition to these policies, many medical schools now provide courses on how to disclose and discuss medical errors with patients. Thus, consider taking such a course so you'll be prepared if you ever find yourself in this *What if* scenario.

Perhaps the best evidence of the advantages of disclosure and apology is a statement by a plaintiff's attorney made to the *Wall Street Journal* in June 2004, "The hardest case for me to bring is the case where the defense has admitted error. If you have no conflict, you have no story, you have no debate, and it doesn't play well."

What if . . .

There is a very bad outcome to a labor and delivery that you were involved with?

This *What if* scenario can happen to you in several ways. The spectrum ranges from a scenario in which you're the physician who did the delivery to a scenario in which a couple that you're friends with has had a stillborn child. If you were the attending physician on the delivery and there were mistakes or errors made, consider a sincere apology and other measures of disclosure as appropriate. (See the *What if* on page 205.) Here, we'll focus more on the scenario in which you aren't the attending physician. Perhaps you're seeing a patient for a nonobstetrical reason, who has recently suffered a fetal death or pregnancy ending in a stillbirth. Or perhaps you are simply meeting a friend who has suffered this loss.

Approximately 6 to 10 births per 1000 are stillbirths. Stillbirths and fetal deaths are obviously traumatic for the parents. It's important to understand the emotions that these parents are experiencing. This event is experienced as a death of their baby and comes with many other difficult emotions, such as a sense of loss of their role as a parent, a loss of a dream, a loss of their confidence in having children, and much uncertainty and despair.

What To Do

You must approach such parents with caring and a desire to understand their loss. They'll want you to understand the depth of their feeling of loss and allow them to express their feelings. Be as supportive as you can. Acknowledge the severity of what they have gone through. Encourage them to talk about what happened. They'll also be trying to understand what happened, to know why it happened, and to know if it will happen again. As a physician, you'll be expected to speak about these subjects with some degree of authority.

Most importantly: Listen. Try to assess their level of understanding. Answer medical questions to the best of your ability. Say you don't know when you don't know. In any of your responses, be careful to be nonjudgmental and don't inadvertently impose feelings of guilt. The range of emotions will include the expected grief and sadness but will also likely include anxiety, anger, denial, and a need to blame. Keep in mind that each of the parents will probably express grief and other emotions differently from the other. Be understanding of this difference and flexible about it.

Most obstetrical units in hospitals have policies and procedures in place for this scenario, including professional counselors to work with the parents. Generally, the staff on the obstetric unit will encourage the mother and father to hold the stillborn infant and name the child. This practice is an established method used to facilitate the grieving process. However, recent studies suggest that mothers who have held the stillborn child have longer periods of grief and subsequent depression. Some parents will refuse to hold or name the stillborn child and this feeling should be respected.

Encourage the couple to seek professional counseling. The parents have much to deal and cope with over the ensuing weeks and months. In addition to accepting the death, they must inform family and friends, perhaps undo home preparations for a new child, possibly deal with the emotions of other children at home, and deal with their own grief.

Be prepared for their questions: How could this happen? What causes a stillbirth or death in utero? Will this happen again? It's wise to recommend an autopsy, even though 50% of the time it doesn't yield a cause of death. The risk of subsequent fetal death or stillbirth is slightly higher in those who have experienced such events in the past, especially if the event occurred at less than 27 weeks of gestation—perhaps as high as 40 to 50 per 1000 births. (After 27 weeks, the risk is much lower—more in the vicinity of 3 per 1000 births.) The couple should be encouraged to have another child if they desire, but to wait until they have accepted and adjusted to this tragic event. Typically, that means they should not attempt a pregnancy for 6 to 12 months after the event.

COPING

How are *you* feeling? Yes, this scenario is hardest for the parents, but be aware that you'll go through parallel feelings of anger, denial, sorrow, depression, or remorse. These feelings are normal under the circumstances. You're human, too. Talk about your feelings with a respected colleague or mentor. Keep in mind that you did everything you could to promote a good outcome. Yes, you'll inevitably think of some things you could have done differently. That's what good physicians do on every case and they learn from those cases. Take solace in knowing that you've been there to help and prepare those parents to the best of your ability.

Prevention and Preparation

Of course, if you were directly involved in the clinical care of the patient, you have done everything possible to cause a good outcome. Unfortunately, despite all those efforts, bad outcomes do happen. You can never prevent someone's feelings of loss or grief. However, with an opportunity for advanced preparation, you may be able to minimize feelings of anger, frustration, or even denial.

If you're involved in the patient's care for some time before the delivery, you may have the opportunity to discuss and educate the patient and her spouse about the risks of the pregnancy, the risks of the planned method of delivery, and the possible poor outcomes. Communication is crucial in good patient care. Speak to the patient about the risks in terms that are understandable to nonmedical people. Typically, the more effective way to describe the possible risks is in events per a number of pregnancies. For example, the risk of dying from a pregnancy and birth is about 1 in 15,000, the risk of fetal loss from amniocentesis is about 1 in 200, and the risk of postoperative infection of the wound is 1 in 15. It sometimes helps to compare a risk to a nonmedical risk, such as the risk of death from a lightning strike is 1 in 10,000.

Finally, take the time to conduct a well-planned informed consent. Disclosure, discussion, and education are valuable for many reasons from a medical-legal point of view, but can also help reduce the severity of bad feelings if a bad outcome does result.

What if . . .

Faraway Adventures

What if . . . You're miles from help on a mountain trail and you or your companion suffers a serious injury?

Most wilderness injuries are caused by:

a. reality television.
b. gangs of surly otters wielding baseball bats.
c. natural disasters.
d. preventable events.

The answer is—d. Proper preparation can prevent most wilderness injuries and help you cope with them when they occur.

What To Do

First, hold off on any assessment until everyone is out of harm's way. Then place anyone injured on level ground protected from the environment and on top of a sleeping bag or clothing that insulates the victim from the ground. Keep all victims warm and dry, removing wet clothing and wrapping them with dry blankets or clothes.

In general, the same principles apply whether you or others are injured. Because there are certain things that you can't do to yourself, such as administer cardiopulmonary resuscitation (CPR), notify others as soon as possible, even if your injuries are seemingly minor. You never know how seriously you've been hurt and when you may fall unconscious or need assistance. Because thorough and objective self-evaluation is difficult, have someone else assess you. If no one else is around, find a mirror or a reflective surface such as water.

Every Breath You Take

Check the ABCs (airway, breathing, and circulation). Administer CPR if necessary. If ABCs are adequate, start assessing from head to toe, looking for injuries—even if the cause, nature, and location of the primary injury is known. Assume a neck injury until you can rule out such an injury. If the patient is conscious, check his neck for signs of injury, such as pain, bruising, bleeding, or deformity. Any evidence of a head injury raises the possibility of a neck injury. If the patient is unconscious, you won't be able to rule out a neck injury.

TO TOURNIQUET OR NOT TO TOURNIQUET?

That is the question. Tourniquets can seriously damage tissue by starving it of oxygen and directly damaging underlying blood vessels and nerves. So, when life-threatening bleeding is occurring, don't use a tourniquet until other methods (such as applying direct pressure, elevating the wound above the heart, compressing the artery that leads to the injury, and using blood-clotting agents or bandages) have failed to stop the bleeding. Once a tourniquet is in place, write down the time it was placed and don't loosen or remove it until the victim has reached medical help.

 WARNING!!! Make sure you search the victim's entire body carefully. Missed injuries can be devastating.

Help?

The next big decision will be whether the injury necessitates transport to emergency facilities and, if so, how far help may be and how mobile the victim is. If the victim can't walk or be transported safely, keep him in place and signal for or seek help.

Message in a Bottle

If you have a cell phone, this would not be the time to worry about roaming and long-distance charges. You must relay your location to the emergency operator, so provide as many landmarks as possible. If you don't have a communication device, then signal for help.

Although Gilligan's Island isn't an ideal model for rescue strategies, some of their signaling techniques may be useful: a large, visible SOS in the sand, a signaling mirror, a flare, a fire, or a beacon. (Just make sure Gilligan doesn't go anywhere near these items.) Remember the number three: three of anything (such as fires, orange flags, whistle blasts, and gun shots) is a universal signal for help, especially when three objects are arranged in a triangle. Choose the most visible areas, such as the top of a hill, to place these signals. Signals visible to flying airplanes may not be as visible to people on the ground and vice-versa. Screaming only works if others are nearby, so don't waste your voice.

Should I Stay or Should I Go?

The toughest decision may be whether to leave the victim to seek help. With more than three people in your group, at least one person can stay with the victim, while others look for help. However, if you're the only other person, then assess the chances of someone spotting your rescue signals, the urgency of the injury, the safety of the current location, and the distance from known available help. For example, if the victim needs help soon, you aren't providing active treatment, assistance is close by, and there's no imminent additional danger, then leaving the victim may be the best choice. If you do leave the victim alone, make sure that he's protected from the elements and surrounded by signaling devices.

BASIC MEDICAL KIT

The basic medical kit should include:

- Basic wound care supplies such as adhesive bandages, gauze, tape, and blister care
- Sunscreen, insect repellent, antibiotic ointment
- Anti-inflammatory or analgesic medications, antihistamines, antidiarrheal medications
- Scissors and forceps
- Water purification devices and supplies

Prevention and Preparation

Preparing for a hike is like preparing for a basketball game:

- **Know the game.** Consult guidebooks, weather forecasts, and people with experience to plan your hike. Locate primary and alternate routes and places to seek assistance. Avoid inclement weather. Bring maps and perhaps a compass or global positioning system (GPS) device.

- **Get the right players.** Your companions should have the right skills, experience, personalities, and amount of emotional and physical stamina. Poor cooperation can be dangerous.
- **Be in shape.** Start training at least 2 months before strenuous hikes. Get evaluated and cleared by appropriate health-care professionals.
- **Bring the right clothing and equipment.** Keep warm, dry, and protected from the elements. Dressing in layers gives versatility and insulation. Synthetic fibers such as polypropylene, rather than natural fibers such as cotton, which doesn't dry as well, may be better for the layer closest to the skin. The outermost layer should be breathable and waterproof. Bring hats, gloves, eye protection, and extra socks. Wear appropriate footwear. Bring a medical kit for longer and more remote hikes. However, don't carry more than you can handle. Pack wisely. After all, being light enough to maneuver safely will allow you to evade any gangs of surly otters with baseball equipment.

> ### BASIC MEDICAL KIT *(continued)*
>
> **Other take-alongs**
>
> Also, consider bringing epinephrine injections for life-threatening allergic reactions and oral antibiotics for soft tissue, respiratory, urinary tract, and gastrointestinal infections. For trips at high altitude, bring medications to prevent and treat altitude sickness.

What if . . .

Your hiking companion suffers a shoulder dislocation?

The shoulder joint, or the *glenohumeral joint,* is the most commonly injured major joint in the body because it has the widest range of motion. It's the junction of three bones: the humerus, scapula, and clavicle. Four muscles and tendons, collectively called the *rotator cuff,* stabilize the humerus in the glenoid, the socket in which the upper arm lifts and rotates. A dislocation occurs when the humerus is forced anteriorly, posteriorly, or inferiorly out of the glenoid by direct force to the joint or weakness of the rotator cuff. More than 95% of shoulder dislocations are anterior.

Certain activities pose a higher risk of dislocations. Any activity where the arm is lifted and twisted, such as throwing or hitting a ball, may dislocate the joint. A direct fall onto an outstretched hand or a backward blow while the shoulder is raised can also force the joint from the socket. People with connective tissue laxity, such as those with Marfan's syndrome, may dislocate a joint with minimal trauma.

A person with a dislocated shoulder may complain of severe shoulder pain, numbness over the deltoid area (axillary nerve damage), and inability to move the shoulder. The extremity is most comfortably held across the body, with the elbow flexed. On examination, the shoulder may appear bruised, swollen, tender, and squared-off compared with the other side.

What To Do

If you suspect that your companion has a shoulder dislocation, gently secure the arm across the chest by slinging a towel underneath the forearm and tying a knot at the nape of the neck near the other shoulder. Even though all displaced joints need to be relocated eventually, only those that cause neurological or vascular compromise need to be reduced immediately. Therefore, you must feel for a radial pulse by palpating the palm side of the wrist near the bottom of the thumb and check nerve function by testing for sensation on the deltoid muscle. If pulse and nerve function are intact, then you can wait for a physician to perform the reduction.

 WARNING!!! If the patient has no pulse, deltoid sensation, or a cold hand, you must reduce the shoulder immediately! With vessel or nerve damage, waiting even 30 minutes may mean losing use of the entire arm.

There are several ways to replace the humerus back into its socket. First, make sure the patient is seated on a flat surface. Then follow one of these three methods:

1. Have your companion walk his fingers slowly up the side of his body past his armpit and ear to touch the top of his head. He should feel a "click" when the shoulder pops back in.
2. If you're traveling with someone else, use him to hold the patient steady while you apply constant force to the patient's arm by pulling it toward the ground. You should feel the shoulder popping back into place.
3. Lift the patient's flexed elbow up toward his head so that he can touch the top of his head. You may feel a "click" when the shoulder pops back into place.

Following each successful reduction, check the pulse and deltoid sensation, then replace the sling to prevent the shoulder from popping out again.

 WARNING!!! Don't force the bones back into place because you could damage the axillary nerve or cause the humerus to break. If you don't know how to relocate the shoulder, make sure it's secured to the body with the sling, and promptly call for help.

WATCH OUT FOR...

Multiple injuries

Any shoulder trauma may be associated with trauma elsewhere on the body, such as the chest wall, which can cause breathing difficulties. Make sure you call for help immediately if you suspect multiple injuries. Leave the scene promptly if there is impending danger.

Prevention and Preparation

There are several ways you can prevent this unintentional shoulder injury. A previously dislocated shoulder joint will be more easily dislocated than an uninjured shoulder, so make sure you strengthen those rotator cuff muscles with exercise. Always wear proper protective gear while exercising or playing sports to guard against inadvertent blows to your shoulder. Furthermore, before you leave the house to go hiking in the woods or walking leisurely through a park, make sure you wear the appropriate shoes for the terrain. Just remember, trying to impress someone by wearing fancy shoes might be sabotaged by an ungraceful fall!

AMATEUR.

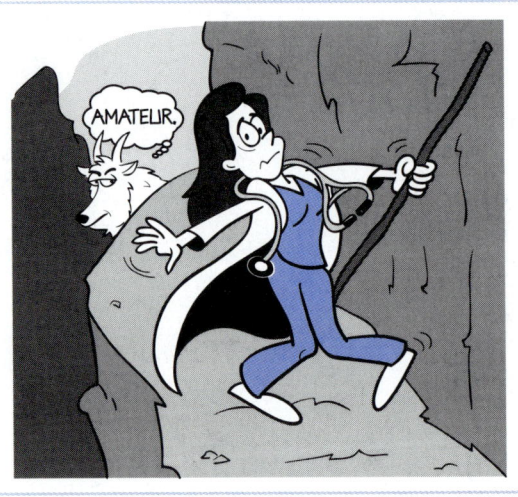

What if . . .

You're hiking or skiing at high altitude and you or a companion shows signs of severe altitude sickness?

It's a common misconception that you can develop altitude sickness only if you travel to exotic places such as Cusco, Peru (11,000 feet) or Lhasa, Tibet (12,500 feet). Several U.S. cities are located at altitudes that might cause altitude sickness as well, specifically the Grand Canyon (6606 feet) and Gunnison, Colorado (7673 feet). Even though serious illness rarely occurs below 9000 feet, you can experience mild symptoms at altitudes as low as 4000 feet, akin to the level of Idaho Falls.

Anyone who goes to a higher altitude will experience certain physiological changes while the body acclimatizes to the lower atmospheric oxygen. Travelers might breathe faster, experience shortness of breath during exertion, and urinate more often. At night, they might wake up more frequently, have strange dreams, and breathe periodically in a Cheyne-Stokes pattern. Anyone—even a young, physically fit person—can develop altitude sickness, especially when the ascent occurs too quickly for acclimatization to occur.

So how would you recognize when someone is starting to get altitude sickness? Well, there are really only three potentially lethal syndromes that you'll need to recognize:

- Acute mountain sickness (AMS)
- High altitude cerebral edema (HACE)
- High altitude pulmonary edema (HAPE).

 WARNING!!! Any illness that occurs at altitude is altitude sickness until proven otherwise. Some people will only get the brain symptoms, whereas others will only get the pulmonary symptoms.

AMS, the most common form of altitude sickness, typically occurs during a rapid ascent. Travelers usually complain of headaches, nausea, vomiting, generalized fatigue, confusion, or difficulty sleeping, much like a bad hangover. They might appear to sway from side to side while walking, like someone who drank too much alcohol at a late-night party. Do NOT simply assume that they drank those beers they snuck into their backpacks or that they're just clowning around.

In HACE, a severe form of AMS, the brain actually swells and stops functioning properly. People with HACE lose the ability to think properly and commonly are very confused, behave strangely, or are lethargic. They'll also stagger around like someone who's intoxicated and actually fall down if they try to walk in a straight line. Mild edema can rapidly progress to severe edema, resulting in brain herniation and death.

In HAPE, another severe form of altitude sickness, the lungs flood with fluid. This condition may also occur in AMS or is seen as a subset of AMS but, as mentioned before, may be seen in the absence of any neurological symptoms. (Neurological symptoms are part of HACE or may be seen with hypoxia to the cerebral blood vessels.) Travelers may have fatigue, shortness of breath at rest, chest tightness or congestion, and cough that produces pink, frothy sputum. They may have cyanotic lips or nailbeds, suggesting a lack of oxygen to their bodies. As with HACE, this condition must be recognized and treated immediately because delaying treatment may be fatal.

What To Do

Recognizing the problem is half the battle; if you don't recognize the illness, you can't treat it. The mainstay of treatment for altitude sickness is to STOP the ascent or quickly DESCEND to a lower altitude.

Stop What You're Doing

If your friend tells you that he has a headache, feels fatigued, or is lightheaded, then you should stay at that same altitude until those symptoms resolve and the body acclimatizes to the atmospheric change. Mild analgesics (such as Tylenol,

THINGS TO REMEMBER

Do's and Don'ts of altitude sickness

Do's

- Assume that any illness that occurs at altitude is altitude sickness until proven otherwise.
- If your symptoms get worse, descend immediately.
- Take the time to properly acclimatize your body to the new altitude. There is no better prevention for altitude sickness.

Don'ts

- Never ascend with any symptoms of altitude sickness, even minor ones.
- Never leave someone with altitude sickness alone.

aspirin, or ibuprofen) and drinking lots of fluids may help relieve the headache. A commonly used medication is acetazolamide, which acts on the kidneys to acidify the blood, balancing the affects of hyperventilation that occurs normally. It doesn't cure AMS immediately, but it does speed up the process. In addition to acetazolamide, dexamethasone, nifedipine, and salmeterol have been used to treat severe disease. Dexamethasone is a steroid medication that can treat AMS and HACE. Nifedipine (an antihypertensive) and salmeterol (an inhaled steroid) are sometimes used to treat HAPE. All drugs should be used carefully, preferably with physician consultation.

Begin Your Descent

Moreover, if you descend to a lower altitude, your friend will get better much faster. Once those symptoms disappear, then it's usually safe to climb again. Similarly, people with severe brain swelling or difficulty breathing must descend immediately to a lower altitude, even if the symptoms develop at night. It can't wait until morning because the person will be unable to walk on his own by then! How far down should you descend? At the very least, you should go to the last elevation at which the person had no symptoms. If you aren't sure when that was, usually it's the elevation where the person slept two nights ago. Another good rule of thumb is to descend about 500 to 1000 meters. Descent will be very difficult and slow-going because the patient will be staggering around acting confused or be breathless and fatigued. Be prepared to carry him if necessary and keep him warm. Just remember that if he doesn't go down, he might die. HACE and HAPE resolve with descent and rest at a lower elevation for a few days. Once the symptoms disappear, your friend may climb again—cautiously.

Prevention and Preparation

There are several ways to prevent severe altitude sickness. Ascend slowly up a mountain and give your body a chance to acclimatize to the atmospheric change. Avoid overexertion and make sure you take time to rest. Always travel in groups so that someone else is available to help you in case you get sick. Avoid using such drugs as alcohol, sleeping pills, and narcotic pain pills, all of which can cause breathing problems and sleepiness. Make sure that you stay hydrated while you climb, because dehydration can worsen symptoms. Finally, preventive medications like acetazolamide may shorten the acclimatization period, which is useful if you're flying to a high altitude (rapid forced ascent) or if you've had mountain sickness in the past. For more information about altitude sickness, check out these websites before you travel:

- Centers for Disease Control and Prevention traveler's website at *www.cdc.gov/travel/diseases/altitude.htm*
- High Altitude Medicine Guide at *www.high-altitude-medicine.com.*

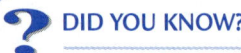 **DID YOU KNOW?**

Latest ideas on using Ginkgo and Viagra

Newer medications are being evaluated to prevent altitude sickness. Ginkgo biloba, an herbal remedy, has been shown in small studies to reduce the symptoms of AMS when taken before ascent. However, there are no studies to date comparing ginkgo to acetazolamide, so newer isn't necessarily better.

Viagra has also recently been shown to prevent HAPE, although again, there isn't enough scientific evidence yet to support it. Other drugs that have been used but have not been proven to work are vitamin E, iron, garlic, and progesterone. Until there is more evidence supporting the use of these other drugs, they aren't currently recommended. So keep your eyes out for more information on the use of these drugs.

What if . . . Your hiking companion says, "I just can't go any farther"?

Here's what not to do. Don't:

- Mock and call your companion a "wimp" or "weakling."
- Keep walking and ignore your companion.
- Take his or her wallet, valuables, or lunch.

There could be a number of reasons why your companion can't go any farther—some trivial, some serious. Your companion could be bored, annoyed, hungry, thirsty, or tired. He could be in dire need of a bathroom break. Maybe it's getting late, and your companion is in danger of missing an appointment or a television show. Your companion could be joking or acting melodramatic.

However, he could be having a serious medical problem that, if overlooked, could lead to major or even fatal injury. While some people may overstate their problems, others may understate them, hoping that their problems will go away or fearing that they'll appear weak or burdensome. Sometimes a person can't exactly pinpoint what is wrong, especially while he's moving.

What To Do

Regardless of your companion's personality or previous behavior, at least initially, take his comment seriously. Make sure that he isn't having a significant medical problem, such as breathing difficulties, lightheadedness, nausea, pain, or weakness. Elicit what exactly is preventing your companion from going any farther. Even if he says, "you and your terrible jokes," make sure it isn't a cover for a more serious problem (and stop telling terrible jokes). Look at your companion, because he may not be able to adequately answer. Does he look unusually pale, sweaty, or wobbly? Find a safe place to stop hiking to give your companion an opportunity to rest and elaborate. Sometimes people will initially deny but then later admit their problems. So be patient, ask each question more than once, and make sure your companion responds to each question. Check if your companion is grasping, holding, or clutching any of his body parts, which may be the source of the problem.

 WARNING!!! Don't continue hiking until you're sure your companion isn't having physical problems. Be overcautious. If you have any suspicion that something is seriously wrong, abort the hike and seek medical help.

Prevention and Preparation

Be in proper mental and physical shape. Bring appropriate equipment. Know, communicate with, and pay close attention to your companion. The better you know your companion, the better you'll be able to recognize when he's in real danger. For example, normally very loquacious companions may become abnormally quiet, cheerful companions may become somber, or aggressive companions may turn passive. People will commonly say that they took their spouses to the emergency room because they "sensed" something wasn't right.

A dangerous or strenuous hike is probably not the best place to bring up emotional or controversial issues. However, you should maintain a relatively open atmosphere during the hike. Your companion shouldn't be afraid to reveal a physical problem or concern. Periodically rest and ask your companion how he's feeling. Maybe your companion will be able to warn you about his impending physical problems . . . or at least your terrible joke-telling.

Notes

MY CLIENT SUFFERS FROM
A POOR PUBLIC IMAGE!

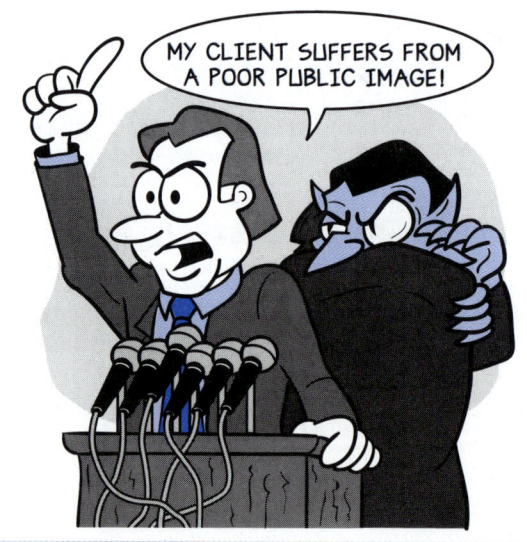

What if . . .

You need to care for a snakebite victim on a mountain trail?

"I hate snakes."

–Indiana Jones in *Raiders of the Lost Ark* and *Temple of Doom*

Thanks to Indiana Jones (and others), snakes suffer from a poor public image and could use the help of a good publicist. Snakes commonly conjure up frightening images of venomous and deadly creatures. As a result, snakebites can be more frightening than bites from most other animals, causing victims to panic and display symptoms such as fainting, gastrointestinal problems, temperature changes, and tachycardia that can easily be misinterpreted as snake venom poisoning. However, in the May 2004 issue of *Emergency Medicine Clinics of North America*, Gold, Barish, and Dart reported that only 15% of the 3000 species of snakes in the world are considered dangerous to humans. According to Jackett and Hancox's April 2002 *American Family Physician* article on snakes, in the United States, less than 20% of the approximately 45,000 annual snake bites are from poisonous species and fewer than 10 to 15 deaths occur each year. Furthermore, 25% to 50% of bites by venomous snakes are "dry" bites and don't result in the injection of venom to the victim. The type and size of the snake, the age and health of the victim, and the location and amount of venom injected into the bite determine the risk. So, although appropriate measures should be taken, you and the snakebitten person shouldn't panic.

In the United States, most venomous snakebites in the wilderness come from the *Crotalidae*, or pit viper family, which includes rattlesnakes, copperheads, and cottonmouths. Some come from coral snakes, members of the *Elapidae* family. Although it's difficult to properly identify snakes, pit vipers have a few distinguishing features, including heat-sensing facial "pits" below each nostril, triangular heads (versus rounded heads), elliptical pupils (versus rounded pupils), and two curved fangs. When aroused, rattlesnakes may vibrate or "rattle" keratin rings at their tail ends to cause a buzzing sound but they can strike without "rattling." Copperhead bites are less toxic than rattlesnake or cottonmouth bites and may not require treatment. Although color variations exist, coral snakes typically have broad, red, yellow (or cream), and black bands. They have short fangs and are nocturnal and usually nonaggressive.

Snake venom consists of enzymes that break down a variety of tissues, including nerves, muscle, blood, and connective tissue. The venom can also trigger blood coagulation disorders that, in turn, can cause damage to many different organs, including the lungs, heart, and kidneys. The first symptoms are usually burning pain, followed by swelling at the bite site. The swelling can be quite variable and even involve the entire limb. Blistering or bruising can also occur. Victims may experience a rubbery, minty, or metallic taste, low blood pressure, rapid heart rate, rapid breathing, nausea, vomiting, tingling, numbness, or mental status changes. Bites that result in only a small amount of venom being injected may only cause local symptoms limited to around the bite site and may not require treatment, aside from close observation and fluids. A larger amount of venom may cause life-threatening problems and require treatment with antivenin.

What To Do

Get you and the victim away from the snake so that neither of you get bitten again. Even dead and decapitated snakes can transfer venom when touched. If you can't see the snake, move the victim to a clear, safe area.

Your goal is to stabilize the victim until he can be brought to a medical facility. Assess the victim and administer emergency cardiopulmonary resuscitation if he isn't breathing. Keep the victim warm, calm, resting, and free of items that may be constricting, such as bands, watches, rings, and tight clothing. Keep the bitten area immobilized and below the level of the heart. Don't give any stimulants, caffeine, or alcohol that may increase blood circulation and the spread of venom. Watch the victim carefully, as signs and symptoms may take up to 12 hours to develop. Remember, even if the patient feels fine, he should be taken to a medical facility as soon as possible.

 WARNING!!! Although seen frequently on television and in movies, sucking out the poison, using tourniquets, applying ice or electricity, or cutting the injured area have NOT been proven to be effective and may introduce bacteria to the wound or cause tissue damage. If someone has already placed a tourniquet, don't remove it unless it's causing damage to the victim's limb.

Prevention and Preparation

Don't try to handle, threaten, or taunt snakes. (If you must taunt or insult snakes, do so in a language or manner they don't understand, such as using elaborate metaphors.) Treat snakes like royalty and give them lots of room to pass, at least 6 feet. Beware of areas that may harbor snakes, such as dense vegetation, firewood, lumber, logs, and rocks. Before walking in such areas, use a long stick or pole to poke suspicious areas and scare snakes away. Wear loose, thick, long pants and tall boots when in snake-infested areas. Most importantly, don't let paranoia of snakes distract you from other wilderness risks. After all, Indiana Jones faced far greater danger from competing relic hunters and film critics.

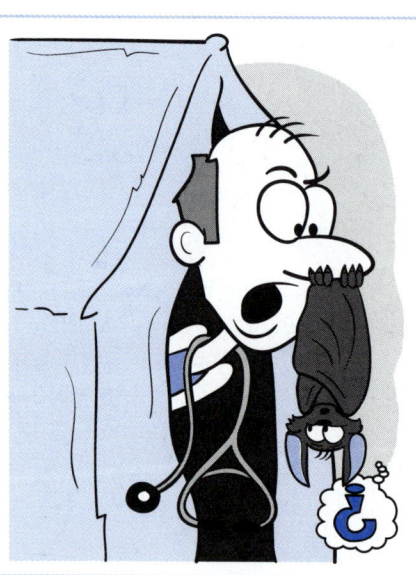

What if . . .

You have a close encounter with a bat?

Having a close encounter with a bat is like waking up after a wild night of overindulgent partying. You know what could have happened, but may not be sure what actually occurred. Everything may be all right. On the other hand, very bad things could have happened.

Bats are a major source of rabies in the United States. Unfortunately, some people who contract rabies from bats can't recall being bitten. Genetic analysis can confirm that the rabies virus indeed came from a bat but, for reasons that are still unclear, not all victims realize how and when they were infected. Perhaps many bat bites are too small to be noticed. Their saliva can transmit rabies if it strikes your eye, nose, mouth, or wounds. There may be additional ways that bats can spread rabies through the air without biting someone. The means by which bats can transmit rabies and the frequency of unnoticed transmissions remain under debate. So every close bat encounter should be taken seriously. If you were asleep, intoxicated, or somehow impaired while a bat was in the room, assume the worst. Once symptoms develop, rabies is fatal with no cure. So have a low threshold for getting treatment with antirabies vaccine or rabies immune globulin (RIG) if you may have been exposed to the rabies virus.

Bats can also transmit histoplasmosis, a fungus, through their guano (i.e., poop). Most people (more than 90%) who contract histoplasmosis have either no problems or just mild symptoms. A small percentage can become seriously ill and potentially die without treatment.

What To Do

Don't panic. (Is there ever a situation when panicking is good?) Call your local county health agency, which can provide instructions and assistance. If possible, trap the bat in a room in a way that doesn't risk another close encounter, so that the bat can be tested for rabies. The county health agency will provide a professional to capture the bat.

If no professionals are available, take appropriate measures to safely catch the bat. Wear a pair of thick leather gloves. Wait until the bat lands, then approach it slowly carrying a box or similar container, and try to trap the bat under the box or container. Slide a piece of cardboard under the container and seal it with tape. Poke some small holes in the cardboard for the bat to breathe and arrange for the bat to be rabies tested with the health department.

Look for bites and clean them extensively with soap and water to prevent bacterial infection. Cleaning with povidone iodine solution or 70% alcohol may reduce the risk of rabies transmission. You must be assessed by medical professionals who will then determine if you need to be treated with rabies vaccine and RIG.

Prevention and Preparation

Keep away from bats. (They don't make very good friends, anyway, since they sleep all day.) Be particularly careful about bats exhibiting unusual behavior such as flying during the daytime, bumping into things, or being unable to fly, signs that they may be rabid. If you absolutely must handle a bat, wear very

? DID YOU KNOW?

Facts about bat rabies

- The virus multiplies in muscle cells near the bite and then travels up peripheral nerves into the central nervous system.
- Symptoms can take a while to develop (most commonly 30 to 90 days, but in some cases several years after exposure).
- Early symptoms may include headache, fever, runny nose, sore throat, muscle aches, GI symptoms, back pain and spasms, agitation and anxiety, and tingling or pain at the bite site.
- There are two types of full-blown rabies—the "furious" and the "dumb"—that may overlap or progress to one

another. In the more common "furious" (or *encephalitic*) form, patients may become extremely agitated and irritable and suffer violent, jerky contractions of the breathing muscles when attempting to swallow liquids, which may contribute to an overwhelming fear of water. In the less common "dumb" (or *paralytic*) form, the symptoms resemble Guillain-Barré syndrome (weakness and tingling followed by paralysis). Ultimately, in both, coma and death occur.

- Once symptoms develop, rabies is commonly fatal within 3 to 10 days. Very few people have survived rabies after symptom development.

thick gloves and cover exposed skin. If you anticipate being frequently exposed to bats (such as an animal handler, a power line worker who has to remove bats, or someone living in an endemic area), get immunized against rabies.

Bat-proof your house by covering all openings with screens. Bats commonly enter through open windows, doors, and vents; under eaves and loose siding; or down chimneys. The best time to do the bat-proofing is during the fall and winter, when bats hibernate. If you find a bat in your house, call a bat-removal expert. (Your county health agency can provide a list of such experts.) Stay away from and seal off the room with the bat. In many cases, the bat may just leave through the opening it came in. One bat may be a sign that others have nested in your house. So search your house carefully.

 WARNING!!! Don't sniff bat poop. (There are certainly better things to do with your spare time.) If you have to clean bat guano (poop), wear a respirator to prevent histoplasmosis or get a professional to clean it.

In general, there is no need to be paranoid. Seeing a bat from afar doesn't constitute a close encounter. Bats are usually not aggressive and can be quite docile. So, if you leave them alone, they'll likely treat you the same way. Just like going out for a night on the town, if you take the proper precautions, moderate your behavior, and enjoy things from a safe distance, you won't find yourself with an unexpected companion (like the bat) that you may have to bring in for further evaluation.

What if . . .

You're lost in the mountains and out of water?

Water is like that important friend who you take for granted until he's gone. Comprising over 70% of our body weight, water is the virtual Renaissance molecule for our bodies, performing a multitude of essential tasks, including catalyzing vital chemical reactions, supporting the architecture of cells, and transporting nutrients and toxins. You may be able to survive for weeks without food, but it's unlikely that you'll survive more then a few days without water. Dehydration will quickly compromise your mental and physical abilities so, next to finding shelter and warmth, finding drinkable water is the most important thing to do when you're lost.

What To Do

Remember, keeping hydrated means more water in AND less water out of your body. So don't expend a lot of energy and perspiration building an elaborate contraption just to get a small amount of water. Don't sacrifice water for food, like chasing after a wild boar, climbing mountains to get edible plants, or eating things that will make you more dehydrated, such as protein bars, potato chips, or French fries.

Purify, Purify

If possible, purify all water before consumption. Although there are many potential sources of water in the wilderness, unless you happen to come across a water cooler or a convenience store, none will be completely clean. Boiling water can effectively kill most organisms. Halogens, such as iodine and chlorine, can work but may be ineffective against *Cryptosporidium*. They may also bind with and be inactivated by solid material in the water or not work at certain temperatures or pH levels. In addition, if the water is cold, it may take longer (more than 30 minutes) for the halogen to disinfect. Filters can remove large organisms, but not viruses and must be kept clean to remain effective.

 WARNING!!! Be careful with iodine if you have a thyroid condition. The thyroid gland normally absorbs and incorporates iodine into thyroid hormone, so increasing iodine intake could cause hyperthyroidism.

Let It Rain

Although all water has some form of contamination, some water will be better than others. The best sources are rainwater and dew. Rainwater is relatively clean and can be caught by containers or taken from uncontaminated puddles. Look for cleaner puddles that have just formed or are located on rocks or large plant leaves. At first glance, dew may not seem to be much, but at dawn and dusk, dew is everywhere, on plants, rocks, and other objects. Sponge the objects with some cloth or similar porous material and wring the moisture into a container or wrap a clear plastic bag over trees or shrubs to catch any moisture that evaporates. Try to keep the moisture from leaking out of the plastic bag by sealing the bag around the tree branches with tape or string. The more leaves, the more dew. So do not waste your time throwing a plastic bag over a leafless tree.

Freshly Frozen

Freshwater snow and ice are also possible sources. Frozen seawater slowly loses its salt and ultimately becomes drinkable. (Otherwise, stay away from seawater, unless you have a way of removing the salt, which will dehydrate more than hydrate you.) Look for signs that the seawater has been frozen for more than a year, such as rounded corners, brittleness, and bluish or black color, or taste the ice to make sure it isn't salty. Make sure you melt any kind of snow and ice before you consume it, since melting it in your mouth or body requires too much energy. Try to melt large amounts of snow or ice in an efficient manner that produces as much water as possible with as little energy expenditure, such as filling a bag or tarp with snow and using either fire or the sun to melt it. Place a container under the bag to catch the water. Of course, the water may taste like smoke or bag, but that would be least of your problems.

Not Just Fish

Freshwater lakes, streams, and brooks are tempting sources, but may have many little things floating or swimming in them, such as bacteria *(Escherichia coli, Campylobacter, Vibrio cholerae, Shigella, Salmonella, Yersinia enterocolitica),* protozoa *(Giardia, Cryptosporidium),* parasites *(Strongyloides, Ascaris, Taenia),* viruses (hepatitis A and E, Norwalk, polio), and toxins. Unless you're considering the spring where they bottle Evian water or are equipped with water purifiers, look for alternative cleaner sources first. In North America, where the most common infectious agents, *Giardia* and *Cryptosporidium,* have incubation times of 1 to 3 weeks (whereas other agents in other parts of the world or in dirtier water may have shorter incubation times), if you have no other alternatives, you may consider taking a risk if you expect to be rescued soon or take antibiotics like ciprofloxacin or Flagyl that can prevent protozoan and bacterial diarrhea.

Prevention and Preparation

Whenever you go hiking, bring enough water—a minimum of 2 quarts of water per person per day and more under hotter or drier conditions or if you are larger, perspire profusely, or have diarrhea. Use clean containers that won't allow leakage, evaporation, or contamination. Remember, water is also needed for general hygiene and wound irrigation. Consider bringing water purification devices if you plan to take a long trip in a remote area. Before hiking, understand the local topography and where to seek water. Remember water is your most important friend, don't leave home without it.

What if . . .

You're stranded overnight or longer?

Regardless of what beer commercials, fashion designers, and electronics manufacturers may tell you, no items are more important to survival than water, warm clothing, and shelter. The previous *What if* scenario (page 239) already talked about how to find water. Next, you should, ideally, be wearing appropriate clothing that keeps you dry and protects you from the cold. So it's now time to focus on how to obtain or build adequate shelter.

Note: The assumption here is that you aren't stranded overnight in a Four Seasons Hotel, a Pebble Beach resort, or a South of France villa. If you are, the next step is to invite all of us over and order room service. Instead, we're assuming that you don't have access to formal shelter. In harsh environments, getting shelter may be even more urgent than finding water, because you may not be able to survive more than a few hours braving the elements.

What To Do

Determine the local environment's biggest threats, and choose your shelter accordingly. In hot climates, heat will be the problem, so shade is imperative. Cold climates require adequate insulation. In tropical climates, shelters should be elevated and enclosed to keep out insects and dampness. Threats may change throughout the day. For instance, in the desert, a flimsy shaded shelter may protect you from the daytime heat, but not the nighttime cold. Unless you're stranded in a Casino in Monte Carlo, wind and rain will always be potential complications.

Location, Location, Location

Avoid potential hazards, such as unstable trees, loose mountainsides, insects, or areas that may flood. Find enough tree cover to protect against the wind and rain, but not so much to block all warming sun rays. If possible, orient your shelter so that it won't be blown down by the wind by pointing the entrance 45 to 90 degrees away from the direction of the prevailing wind.

Rent, Lease, or Build

Should you use an existing natural shelter, modify a natural shelter, or build a shelter from scratch? Strike a balance between obtaining appropriate shelter and conserving your time and energy. The shelter must be safe from the environment, disturbance-free enough to rest and sleep and, if necessary, conspicuous for rescue and search crews to find. Ensure that there are no unwanted room-

---

MODEL HOMES

Here are some examples of shelters you may construct:

- **Tents and Teepees:** There are lots of variations of tents and teepees. You'll need a sturdy, geometrically stable foundation like trees or poles firmly planted in the ground to either suspend a rope or directly support a canvaslike covering.
- **Debris Hut:** This hut is somewhat similar to the huts seen on Gilligan's Island. Use sticks and poles to create a latticework skeleton of a hut. Then cover the skeleton with layers of debris like grass, pine needles, and leaves.

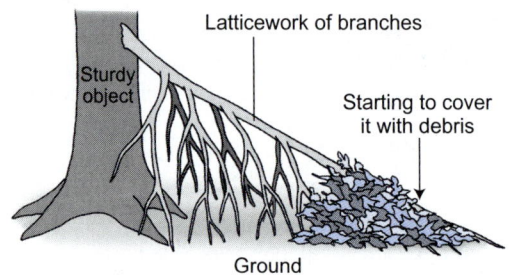

Latticework of branches

Sturdy object

Starting to cover it with debris

Ground

- **Tree-Pit Snow Shelter:** For this shelter, you'll need to find an evergreen tree with lots of bushy branches that can serve as a room. Dig out the snow around the evergreen tree trunk to create a pit to hold you. Pack the snow around the top of and inside the hole. You can find or cut boughs from other evergreen trees to cover the pit and provide additional roofing.

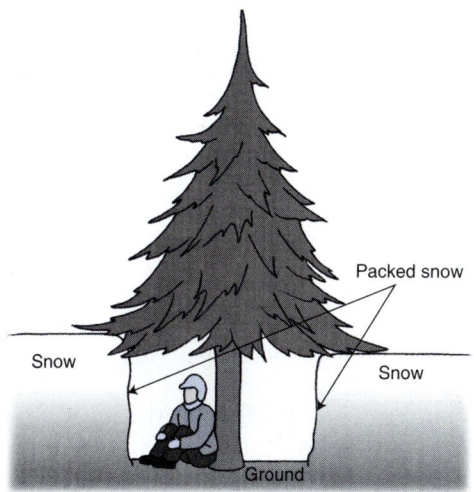

Packed snow

Snow

Snow

Ground

- **Beach Shade Shelter:** This shelter is similar to building a sand castle. Digging a trench while also piling up soil or mud around the trench to make walls can create a structure large enough to hold you. You can then cover the top of the structure with driftwood, layers of leaves or branches, or similar material to form a roof.

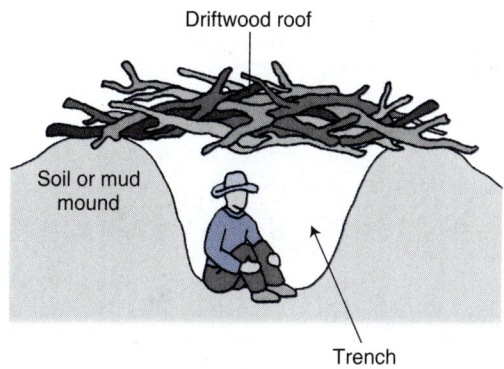

Driftwood roof

Soil or mud mound

Trench

mates, such as bats, insects, rats, snakes, poisonous plants, and vicious reality show contestants. The shelter naturally should be large enough to fit you and your companions, small enough to keep warm and, preferably, have a flat sleeping surface.

Many potential shelters are, like a good face lift, not initially obvious, but can be found with some careful looking and ingenuity. Throwing a covering over two fallen logs, partially blocking off a crevice on the side of a cliff, and digging a hole under an evergreen tree are just some of the ways you can make the landscape into something.

Don't Be Grounded

Direct contact with the ground can lead to heat loss (in cold environments) or absorption (in hot environments). So cover the floor with blankets, clothing, leaves, or pine needles. In hot environments, stay above the ground on a platform or in a hole at least 18″ below ground level. A platform also keeps you drier in wet environments. Stuffing every opening with insulating material helps keep the heat, cold, and critters out. However, maintain at least two openings for ventilation.

LIVING IN A MATERIAL WORLD

Don't have building materials? Look around you for:

- large objects like trees and boulders that can form the walls and foundations of your shelter.
- blankets, ponchos, parachutes, canvas, and plastic bags that can provide covering. (*Note:* Stretch porous material to close off the pores and decrease permeability, and angle shelter roofs at 40° to 60° so rain won't accumulate.)
- rafts, vehicles, or airplane parts that can be used for covering, walls, or other uses.
- rope, string, twine, or vines, to bind materials together.
- other natural materials, such as mud, packed snow, dry moss, leaves, and grass that, when arranged in overlapping layers, can provide waterproofing and insulation.

Prevention and Preparation

Naturally, plan your trips so that you won't get stranded. Study the natural landscape and environment to anticipate potential threats and shelters. Bring shelter building equipment, such as rope or twine, a knife, a digging tool, and covering material such as a tarp. Consider bringing something that can safely heat the shelter, like a battery-operated portable heater. Most importantly, remember, even when the weather seems nice and the only critters around are your companions, having shelter can do wonders for your well-being and, ultimately, your will to survive. Now isn't that worth more than a good beer?

Notes

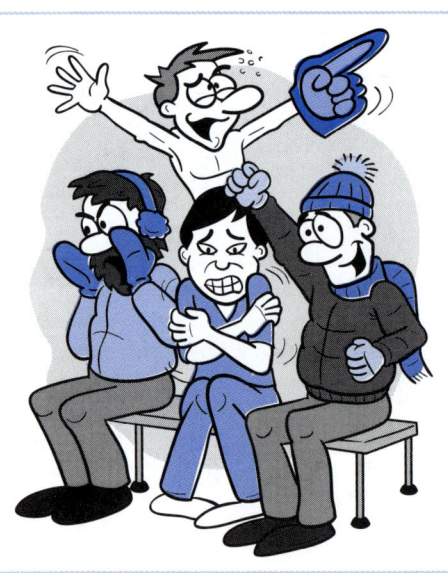

What if . . .

You're getting frostbite?

Frostbite. It's the occupational risk of every Polar Bear Club member, cold weather streaker, and Green Bay Packers fan. There are milder forms of cold injury: pernio (chilblains) from repetitive damp cold exposure, and frostnip, an early, easily reversible form of frostbite.

However, once tissue damage occurs, you have frostbite. In frostbite, the cold destroys skin tissue directly (by freezing the exposed tissue) and indirectly (by disrupting normal blood flow to the tissue). The cold initially interrupts the blood supply to the area by causing blood vessels to constrict, which starves the tissue of oxygen. When the skin thaws, the blood vessels dilate, reestablishing the blood supply. When the blood rushes back into the area, further tissue damage is caused, called *reperfusion injury*. Every time the skin freezes and thaws, more injury occurs. Like burns, frostbite can be superficial (first- and second-degree) or deep (third- and fourth-degree). As skin tissue dies (and, therefore, can no longer be saved), it darkens and becomes harder.

Suspect frostbite if you notice changes in the color, texture, or elasticity of your skin or experience numbness, stinging, or burning. Excessive sweating or clumsiness can also be clues. Frostbite most commonly affects the hands and feet but also occurs on the shins, cheeks, nose, ears, and corneas.

What To Do

Protect the frostbitten area, which is particularly susceptible to damage, by carefully wrapping and padding it with soft, dry clothing or blankets.

 WARNING!!! Avoid rubbing, bumping, or excessively heating the frostbitten area. Don't start rewarming (thawing) the area until you're away from the cold and are sure that the area won't freeze again. Don't drink alcohol or take sedatives as they may worsen heat loss.

Although it should be done promptly, rewarming must be done carefully. Place the area in warm water, (40°C to 42°C), until thawing is complete. Temperatures below this range may not rewarm quickly enough to save all the tissue. Temperatures above this range may cause more damage. Don't use dry heat because the frostbitten area is numb and may not sense the heat until it's burned. Rewarming is complete when blood flow resumes to the area, as evidenced by the return of the normal ruddy blush. Complete thawing typically takes 15 to 30 minutes. After thawing, keep the area elevated, clean, protected, and immobilized.

You should go to the nearest emergency room as soon as possible. Even if thawing was accomplished before getting to the emergency room, physicians will need to care for your wounds, administer antibiotics, and remove any dead tissue. They can also give you pain medications and a tetanus shot if needed.

Prevention and Preparation

Restricting your streaking or Polar Bear activities to warm weather climes like Hawaii, San Diego, or Miami will certainly prevent frostbite. If you must go into the cold, protect yourself by wearing adequate amounts of dry, nonconstrictive, layered clothing, and a warm hat, because your body loses a lot of heat through the head. Minimize the amount of skin you expose by wearing gloves and scarves. Eat and drink adequately to help your body generate heat. Avoid habits that cause heat loss, such as smoking and drinking alcohol or caffeine. Prolonged exposure to temperatures below freezing and even short exposures to extremely cold temperatures will put you at risk.

Finally, heed the warning signs that your body is losing too much heat. So if you're sitting at Lambeau Field (the Green Bay Packers stadium) and you start shivering or feeling numb, take a break from the cold, before it's too late.

Notes

I GUESS YOU'LL WANT THAT AS A MULLIGAN...
18

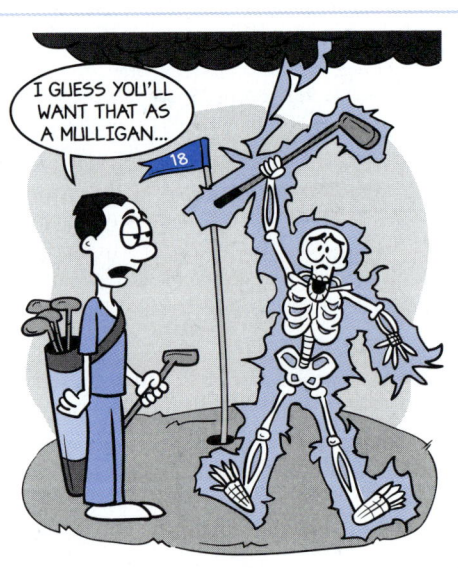

What if . . .

Your friend is struck by lightning?

Many people do survive lightning strikes. Although a lightning strike can deliver a tremendous amount of electricity, intense burning heat, and powerful shock waves that can injure and even throw large objects, it isn't universally fatal. In fact, unless you actually witnessed lightning hit, confirming a lightning injury can be difficult. Amnesia, confusion, or other resulting mental disturbances may prevent victims from remembering or relaying what happened. Featherlike burns on the victim are definitive proof. Exploded clothing, linear burns, ruptured eardrums, and confusion are important clues.

What To Do

In many ways, a lightning strike is similar to any other emergency situation. After making sure the area is clear of danger, determine if the victim needs cardiopulmonary resuscitation (CPR) by checking her consciousness, breathing, and pulse. If necessary, administer CPR promptly and call 911. Keep the victim warm and dry to prevent hypothermia.

Attempt resuscitation on all victims, even those with dilated pupils. Because hypothermia can cause a state that appears like death, warm the victim to nor-

Types of lightning injury

Although lightning was Ben Franklin's friend, it can have a surly disposition and cause lots of bodily damage. Compared to exposure to high voltage electricity, lightning contains more power but typically has a much briefer exposure time, reducing the risk of internal damage.

Burn, break, and throw
Lightning can severely burn the skin and cause fractures of the skull, ribs, spine, arms, or legs. Even without severe burns, the skin can become discolored, as blood flow and temperature control may be disrupted. Weakness, muscle aches, and swelling are common. Although rare, severe damage to the muscles can occur, resulting in the release of muscle proteins that may injure the kidneys (rhabdomyolsis). Moreover, victims may be thrown by the lightning bolt, causing additional trauma.

Strike at the heart
Lightning can also cause a variety of abnormal heart rhythms and even stop the heart from beating. Victims can suffer high blood pressure, a heart attack, or even cardiac death.

Rattle the head and nerves
Headaches, seizures, dizziness, confusion, amnesia, or loss of consciousness can all occur as a result of lightning strike. Mood, sleep, and movement disorders and diffi-

mal body temperature before stopping resuscitation attempts. Major problems may be insidious or delayed, therefore, *all* potential victims should be fully evaluated in the emergency room.

Prevention and Preparation

Although you can never predict when and where a bolt of lightning will strike, to prevent being struck:

- **Listen to your weatherperson.** Staying inside all the time may help prevent lightning strikes, but is impractical and may do irreparable damage to your social life. Instead, keep updated on weather reports and take thunderstorm warnings seriously. Avoid outdoor activities during thunderstorms and seek shelter when the storm approaches.

culty speaking or comprehending other people can begin any time after the lightning strike and persist for days. Lightning can also temporarily or permanently damage the spinal cord, causing paralysis.

Sore eyes . . . and ears
Swelling, bleeding, or permanent damage to the eyes and ears from lightning strike can manifest in perforated eardrums, ringing of the ears, temporary or permanent deafness, transient blindness, or cataracts.

Endanger baby
In pregnant victims, lightning may also be fatal to the fetus.

Host of problems
In general, lightning victims may look like people who have suffered a stroke, a heart attack, head and body trauma, burns, an explosion, or poisoning, all serious problems that require medical attention.

Just a memorable story
Some people come through lightning strikes with minimal or no problems, but everyone still must be properly evaluated by medical personnel as major problems can be hidden or delayed.

- **Listen to the thunder.** Remember, you don't need rain to have thunder and lightning. Some lightning strikes have occurred on reportedly clear days. The shorter the time between seeing a bolt of lightning and hearing the thunder, the closer the lightning bolt. So, if that time is under 30 seconds, the lightning is too close for comfort.
- **Seek adequate shelter.** Tents, cars without solid metal tops, isolated trees, and very small structures aren't adequate shelter. Very small structures may actually be more dangerous. A big building is ideal. A closed, all-metal vehicle can be adequate. Groups in the open should separate to minimize the number of people affected by a strike.
- **Don't show any metal or be wet behind the ears.** Metal and water conduct electricity very well. Drop and avoid larger metal objects (for example, bicycles, fences, tent poles, and golf clubs). Stay clear of the water. Standing close to any water, even dripping water, can be dan-

gerous. If you're in a boat, get out of the open water. Protect your boats with lightning rods and grounding equipment. Moving your boat under a bridge or an overhanging cliff may help.

- **Get shorty.** Being taller is bad; so get off those stilts, get down from that chair, and remove any extensive headgear. If you're outside, squat while covering your ears to protect your eardrums from shock waves. Those who can't squat should kneel or sit cross-legged. Don't lie down; increasing ground contact increases your risk because the ground conducts electricity as well.
- **Don't hold all calls.** Once inside, avoid touching the telephone, sink, bathtub, radiator, pipes, or any electrical appliances or equipment. Stay away from windows, doors, and the fireplace.

Prep Part

With these measures, you may be safer—but not completely safe. So learn and stay up-to-date on your CPR skills. And, if anyone ever tells you that she has been struck by lightning, even if that person was indoors or the sky is clear, take it seriously. You never know . . .

What if . . .

Your friend suffers a fracture on a mountain trail?

Although Humpty Dumpty couldn't be put back together again, you should be able to manage this with just a little instruction. Most importantly, fractures are usually caused by direct trauma to the body, so concurrent injuries are common. Moreover, the patient shouldn't be moved (unless the immediate environment is unsafe) and should be kept as warm and dry as possible. Injury can happen several ways on a mountain trail, such as from falling or sliding, being attacked by an animal, or being struck by a falling branch or tree. Broken bones aren't only painful, but potentially life threatening. Rib fractures may puncture the heart or lungs and cause cardiac or pulmonary contusion, pericardial effusion (blood around the heart), or pneumothorax (air outside the lungs but within the thoracic cavity). Skull fractures may be associated with a brain contusion or intracranial hemorrhage. Pelvic and extremity fractures may cause significant blood loss.

What To Do

In order to properly manage a fracture, you must first recognize it. If it doesn't hurt, it probably isn't broken. Take a good look at the site of injury by comparing it with the equivalent uninjured part. If the skin overlying the injured area is intact, you might see a reddish or bluish discoloration, swelling at the site, obvious deformity, ease of bony movement where there shouldn't be any, a grating sound or sensation with each movement, or inability to bear weight (if legs are involved). Make sure you check for the presence of a pulse, sensation, and movement distal to the injured area. If the overlying skin is torn or cut (an open fracture), you might see exposed bone or actively bleeding vessels. Try not to move the bone fragments too much to avoid more blood loss. Immediately apply direct pressure to stop the bleeding.

Thank goodness we learn the alphabet in kindergarten, because initial stabilization of an injured person follows the ABCDE algorithm:

- Once you're certain that the scene is safe, make sure the **A**irway is cleared of vomit, blood, or broken teeth.
- If the patient isn't **B**reathing, provide rescue breaths.
- Check for any injury to the injured area's **C**irculation by feeling for pulses or controlling active bleeding. If you don't feel a pulse, start CPR.
- Check for any **D**isabilities, such as inability to move an extremity. Make sure you also hold the head still until you can be sure that the person has no spine injuries.
- **E**xpose the patient to identify concurrent injuries and remove clothing that is wet, cold, or contaminated and jewelry that might be too tight.

Open or Closed

In general, fractures are classified as *open* (when the overlying skin is torn) or *closed* (when the overlying skin is intact). Any open injuries should be cleaned and disinfected by rinsing with at least a liter of water, purified with iodine tablets, if possible. Try to realign the bone fragments if they're really angulated or deformed and immediately immobilize the area with a splint. Cover wounds with clean gauze or bandage or use a ripped shirt if necessary to prevent further contamination and infection. Elevate the fractured area to reduce the swelling and, if possible, administer antibiotics if you're several hours from the nearest hospital. Closed fractures are managed according to the injured site:

- *Skull, neck, or back injuries:* These injuries may cause irreversible, devastating neurologic damage because the brain and spinal cord may be concurrently injured. Make sure that your friend is lying flat on the

IMPROVISING SPLINTS

- *Neck splint:* Stuff a medium to large sack about one-quarter full with clothing and slide the flat part of the sack under your friend's neck, resting the stuffed part against one side of the neck. Fill the other side of the sack with clothing so that the neck and head are nestled between the two stuffed ends. Pull the sack closed and secure it to the litter with tape or rope.
- *Pelvic splint:* Pelvic splints are constructed similarly to neck splints, except that they need to be large enough to wrap around the patient's hips. Make sure the hips and the legs are nestled between the two stuffed sections of the sack and secure the sack to the litter.
- *Upper arm splint:* Gather enough rigid material to extend from the shoulder to the elbow and anything that may be used to secure the splint to the arm (such as tape, pack straps, belts, bandanas, and clothing). You may cut your sleeping bag to this length and roll it or fold it over to increase rigidity or use tent poles, trekking poles, or pack frames. Place the splint against the upper arm with the elbow bent at 90° and secure the splint above and below the fractured site. Make a sling by cradling the forearm in the middle of a long piece of clothing and tying the two ends across the opposite shoulder.
- *Lower arm splint:* Gather enough material to extend from the fingers to the elbow. Secure the splint above and below the fracture, keeping the elbow flexed at 90 degrees. Place a wad of cloth in the hand to maintain it in the position of function. Keep the arm loose to the body in a sling.
- *Lower leg splint:* Gather enough material to extend from the hip to the heel on the inside and the outside of the leg. Secure the splint above and below the fracture site.

ground, holding the neck as still as possible. You'll need to call for assistance to get your friend quickly to the nearest medical facility. To move the patient, you must logroll by keeping your friend's head and spine in-line. You'll also need to construct a special litter with a neck splint to transport your friend down the mountain.

- *Chest wall injury:* As previously mentioned, clavicular or rib injuries may puncture the heart or lungs. Don't try to realign any bony fragments because you may cause more injury to the organs underneath. If it's an open fracture, wash the area with water and keep it covered.
- *Pelvis injury:* A lot of force is required to fracture the pelvis, so there's a high risk of concurrent injuries. Pelvic fractures may cause severe internal bleeding, so you must immediately immobilize the pelvis.

YOU SUFFER THE FRACTURE

If you're traveling alone and suffer a fracture, all of the same rules apply. Move to a safe environment, call for help, and carefully assess your injuries. Apply direct pressure to stop any active bleeding. Wash out all open injuries and cover them. You should splint and immobilize any fracture sites. If you suspect a spine injury, call for help, lie down on your sleeping bag, and try to keep your head and back in line while you wait for assistance. Moving around may worsen your spine injury and cause irreversible damage.

Remember, you'll never have to manage these injuries alone if you make sure you always travel with someone.

Your injured friend should lie flat on the ground, without moving too much. As with spine injuries, you should logroll the patient onto a litter for transport.

- *Extremity injury:* Unlike the mentioned injuries, extremity fractures may occur without any injury to an internal organ and aren't usually immediately life-threatening. Any open fractures must be cleaned with water and covered. Remove any constricting jewelry or watch. Any angulated or displaced bony fragments should be realigned by pulling traction on the fragment farthest from the body and sliding it back into place. Remember to check circulation, sensation, and movement distal to the fracture. To reduce the swelling, elevate the extremity above the heart and apply an ice pack to the area. Keep the fracture immobilized.

Prevention and Preparation

Although not all fractures are limb- or life-threatening, it's important to rapidly identify those other potentially dangerous injuries and suppress your inclination to focus all your attention on the obviously injured area. Avoid being out in the wilderness alone because you never know when you might be injured. Consider bringing along a first-aid kit, even on short trips, that includes gauze pads and bandages as well as bottled water, scissors, safety pins, "crazy glue," and additional clothing to add another layer of warmth when necessary. What's more, be on the lookout for potential hazards and warn your hiking partners of any that you see. A high level of alertness, preparation, and communication can help prevent this *What if* from becoming a reality.

Notes

EMERGENCY ROOM
PIZZA

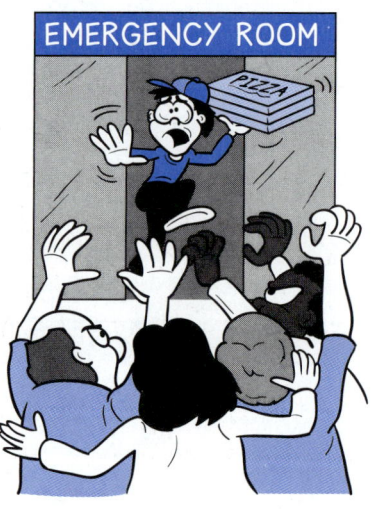

What if . . .

You're trapped by an avalanche?

An avalanche is like a throng of hungry medical students who see a pizza delivery. First, there's a massive rush, then there is a slow down period, and finally everything stops. The key to surviving both events is to recognize the warning signs (such as pizza boxes arriving), brace yourself properly, and wait for the right moment to escape. Trying to escape too soon or too late can spell doom.

What To Do

The Initial Rush

If you see an avalanche, drop all your extraneous equipment: skis, snowshoes, snowmobiles, and tuning forks. Hide behind and hold onto a stable, solid object, such as a large rock or tree. (No, medical textbooks, though generally large, aren't stable enough.) Crouch down, turn away from the avalanche, and brace yourself as the avalanche may tear you away from the solid object and throw you off a cliff, into a tree, or over rocks. Keep your mouth and nose covered, and protect your eyes.

If you're in a car, turn it off immediately to conserve breathable air and minimize the chance of the vehicle exploding or careening off uncontrollably. Close all windows and doors.

The Slowing

Don't do anything else until the avalanche slows. Then, before the avalanche material stops and sets in place, use your arms and hands to clear the material away from your face to create and maintain a breathable air space and then use your legs and torso to "swim" toward the surface. If you've been flipped around, sunlight and less densely packed snow may mark the direction of the surface. The closer you stay to the surface and side of the avalanche while it's in motion, the less you'll have to travel to safety when everything grinds to a halt.

Full Stop

Stay calm. Panicking may waste valuable energy, interfere with your breathing, and bury you further. Dig toward the surface. Use signaling or communication devices, if possible, and call out for rescuers to locate you.

If you're buried in a car, carefully open the window and probe with a pole or stick to determine your depth. If you're close to the surface or don't anticipate help arriving soon, you may venture outside the car. Otherwise, stay in the car, keep the engine off, and use the horn to attract rescuers.

The Aftermath

If you escaped the avalanche, make sure that the avalanche has truly stopped and no other avalanches can occur before trying to locate the other victims. You may be their only hope. First, check for signals, such as avalanche beacons, cries for help, or other noises. If there are none, start "probing": poking long rods, like ski poles, into the snow. Don't worry about accidentally poking the victims. It is far better to be poked by a pole than perish in an avalanche.

Start with high-yield areas, such as downhill from where the victims were last seen and where large amounts of avalanche material accumulated. Be systematic in your searching, marking where you've already probed and covering the area in a gridline. If you have a team of people, you can form a probe line, where everyone stands in a line side-by-side, about 30″ (75 cm) apart, with hands on hips and elbows touching. The leader then tells each person to probe the area at his feet. When everyone is finished, the leader orders the line to advance uphill a short distance, maintaining the straight line, and then probe again in the new location. If someone in the probe line finds a possibility, a few rescuers should dig in the area while the probe line continues its search uphill. The possibility may be a false lead, and there should be no delay in searching for other victims.

 WARNING!!! To avoid injuring or further burying the victim, don't dig too close to or uphill from the victim. Always throw snow downhill; otherwise, you may find yourself in a loop of digging and reburying.

As a general rule, the hole to remove the victim should be as wide as the victim is deep. So if the victim is 10′ below the surface, a 10′-by-10′ hole will be required. Try to expose the victim's head and chest first. Once you have done so, start administering first aid if necessary. Uncovering the rest of the body can wait.

The only reason to abandon buried victims is to avoid immediate danger or get nearby help. If you must leave, post clear markers for you and rescuers to find the area again. Rescuers will also need to know the exact time and location of the accident, the number of victims and other rescuers, and the type of weather conditions and potential routes to the site.

Prevention and Preparation

Before skiing, snowboarding, mountain climbing, or doing anything on a mountain, check the weather forecast or contact the nearest ski patrol or U.S. Forest Service Snow Ranger. If possible, choose slopes that face the wind (windward slopes) and have more trees and rocks for shelter. Cross slopes at their highest points. When your hiking team crosses a risky area, do so one at a time, so that the rest of the team can watch for danger and rescue the person. Carry an avalanche cord, section probe, and avalanche beacon. And, whatever you do, don't stand between pizza and hungry medical students.

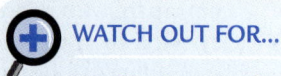

WATCH OUT FOR...

Predicting avalanches

When skiing, snowboarding, or mountain climbing, look for these warning signs

Once, twice, three times an avalanche
- Previous avalanche
- Scars on surrounding trees (suggests prior avalanche)

Weather or not
- Winds of 15 mph or faster
- Rapidly changing temperature
- Snowfall greater than 1″ per hour

Snow thyself
- Soft, new snow greater than 1′ deep
- Dry, loose snow
- Layer of new snow over old snow
- Smaller snow crystals (like needles and pellets)

Express terrain
- Steeper slopes
- Convex slopes (versus concave slopes)
- Slopes that don't face the wind (no wind to blow away and compact loose snow)
- Smooth slopes without large rocks or dense vegetation to anchor snow

What it's cracked up to be
- Cracks in the snow
- Snow that sounds hollow underneath

Notes

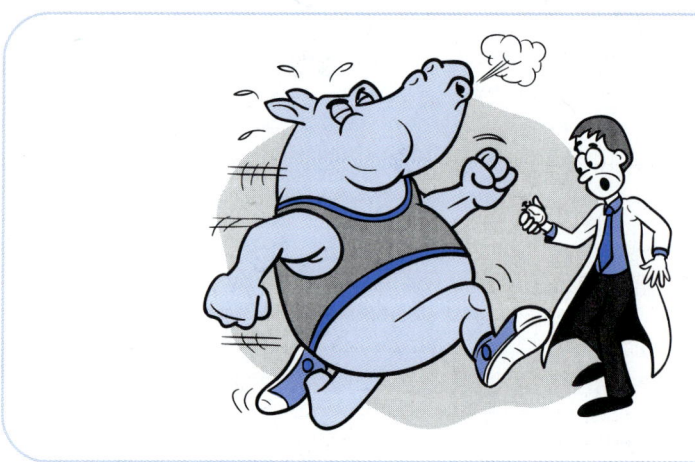

What if . . .

Your friend is attacked by a wild animal?

Wild animals may look cute and cuddly, especially in Disney books and cartoons, but they can do a lot of damage when they attack: inflicting wounds; tearing tissue; breaking bones; puncturing organs; and transmitting infections by biting, clawing, throwing, dragging, and thrashing. Many are faster, stronger, nimbler and, in many ways, smarter (since you are in their element) than you.

What To Do

First and foremost, get you and your friend to safety. How you escape an animal attack depends on what animal and why the animal is attacking. If the animal feels threatened and attacks in self-defense, then gestures that make you seem less threatening, like slowly backing away or lying down protecting yourself, may help. Allow the animal an escape route.

 WARNING!!! When an animal from certain predatory species (such as a mountain lion) attacks, aggressively fighting back may be better than lying down or trying to seem less threatening. Fighting back may actually scare away the animal.

Many animals may be surprisingly tough to outrun. (Picture again a hippo sprinting at 45 miles per hour.) So, finding a safe area to hide, in some cases, may be your best option. (Because detailed instructions on how to escape each type of animal is beyond the scope of this book, consult local wildlife service authorities or animal experts for instructions, especially when heading into the wild.)

When you're safe, check for deep injuries to vital structures, since teeth, claws, horns, or violent impact can puncture, tear, or break major arteries, airways, or organs. If a big cat attacks, be especially vigilant of neck injuries. Resuscitate your friend if necessary. Stop bleeding by applying pressure with a clean bandage or towel. Irrigate and clean wounds with large amounts of clean water and antibacterial solutions, if available. Gently use a soft, clean cloth to remove dirt and foreign objects from the wounds. Dry and cover the wounds with sterile (or as clean as possible) dressings.

Promptly transport your friend to an emergency facility. If help is far away, giving oral antibiotics like amoxicillin-clavulanate, azithromycin, or ciprofloxacin (if available) is reasonable. Immobilize any part of the body where movement may cause further damage (such as broken bones, wounds of the hands or feet, and neck injuries).

Capturing the attacking animal for examination may be helpful, especially if you suspect rabies. Only properly trained individuals should attempt capture, so enlist the aid of forest rangers or other wildlife service authorities, if possible.

? DID YOU KNOW?

Attack modes

Different wild animals use different modes of attack:

- Big cats such as lions, tigers, and cougars, like to attack from behind and bite the victim's head and neck.
- Bears inflict injury with their teeth, claws, and paws.
- Alligators use their jaws and tail to crush the victim's torso and extremities and may roll and drown the victim under water.
- Big birds, such as ostriches, cassowary, and emus (but not Big Bird from *Sesame Street*) kick the victim's head and abdomen, penetrating bodies with their sharp toenails and claws, and peck with their beaks.
- Buffaloes hook victims, toss them in the air, and gore them when they're on the ground.

Prevention and Preparation

If you leave them alone and keep your distance, most wild animals are too busy foraging, resting, thinking, socializing, philosophizing, or scratching themselves

- Elephants can trample or use their tusks to gore and their trunks to strike or throw victims.
- Hippos can easily chop things in half with their large canine teeth and can run up to 45 miles per hour, trampling victims.
- Pigs bite and gore their victims.
- Moose and rhinos charge when they attack.
- Skunks spray secretions that irritate the skin and eyes and can even cause convulsions and loss of consciousness.
- Primates can bite and transmit a host of infectious diseases, including many kinds of bacteria and herpesvirus.
- Porcupines protect themselves with their quills, which can deeply embed themselves in victims and move deeper when the victim moves.

to attack you. Since you can't understand and anticipate their thoughts, behavior, and feelings, approaching them may inadvertently provoke them. Like humans, wild animals are territorial, and walking through the wilderness is like trespassing through their homes and rooms and, not surprisingly, may alarm and threaten them. (What would you do if you found a grizzly bear watching your television or stinking up your bathroom?)

Before you hike in the wilderness, familiarize yourself with the behavior of wild animals that you may encounter and consult experts on how to deal with each species. Never corner an animal or threaten its young. In fact, if you see a mother with her young, stay clear, because you know how protective mothers can be of their children. Get out of the path of moving animals, for they may not see or alter their direction for you. (Once again, picture a hippo moving at 45 miles per hour.) Be especially wary of animals acting oddly (such as walking into things, limping, being unusually aggressive or docile) because they may have rabies or be trying to sell you something. Finally, be careful about exposing food. Smelling like a gigantic hot dog or hamburger may attract unwanted visitors. Keep food concealed and well-wrapped.

However, don't start having nightmares and visions of Big Bird kicking you and hippos sprinting. Most animals will attack only as a last resort and can be safely enjoyed at a reasonable distance. Just remember, you're in their house now.

What if . . .

You or a friend gets a jellyfish sting?

Jellyfish can sting when they come in contact with humans. Jellyfish tentacles are covered with stingers, or *nematocysts,* which release toxins that disrupt cells, interfere with ion transport mechanisms, and release inflammatory mediators. These reactions can lead to a range of symptoms, including a painful rash (common), systemic reactions (occasional), and cardiovascular collapse and death (rare). Nematocysts remain active and can still cause injury for weeks after the animal is dead or even after detachment of the tentacle from the organism.

What To Do

Remove the victim and yourself from the water. Jellyfish sting victims are at risk for drowning. If you see one jellyfish, you know there will be more. It will be harder or maybe impossible to provide assistance if you, too, become a victim. If you become a victim, follow the instructions provided as best you can, or if possible, get assistance from an unaffected companion.

Emergency on-site treatment always begins with the ABCs: airway, breathing, and circulation monitoring. Definitive treatment consists of nematocyst deactivation, pain control, and supportive systemic care:

- *Nematocyst deactivation*—Immobilize the affected area to minimize the uptake of venom. Vigorously rinse the wound with saltwater or seawater and then soak it in vinegar (acetic acid). These two actions inhibit further discharge by unfired nematocysts. Any residual tentacles may be removed using forceps or strong adhesive tape such as duct tape.

 WARNING!!! DON'T rinse the area with fresh or tap water and DON'T rub the skin with a towel or other material usually used to dry off because tap water or mechanical trauma to the nematocysts causes them to rupture and release their toxins into the skin.

- *Pain control*—Cold compresses or ice packs are excellent for relieving pain. Oral pain relieving medications are also helpful. Remember to avoid contact with fresh water as it may activate any remaining nematocysts.
- *Systemic supportive care*—An antihistamine such as Benadryl should be administered to provide supportive care for systemic reactions. Remember, jellyfish sting victims are at risk for anaphylaxis.

Prevention and Preparation

To prevent a jellyfish sting, you may want to avoid swimming in the waters of northern Australia (which would also help you avoid sharks and other dangerous marine animals at the same time!). At any rate, be mindful when swimming in areas with high concentrations of jellyfish. Remember, detached tentacles lying on the beach may still cause envenomations. Rescuers should always wear protective clothing and gloves to protect themselves and better treat the victim. Some experts recommend a sunblock product that inhibits jellyfish stings by blocking the firing of nematocysts. Proper protection and awareness of danger are the best prevention for this *What if* scenario.

Notes

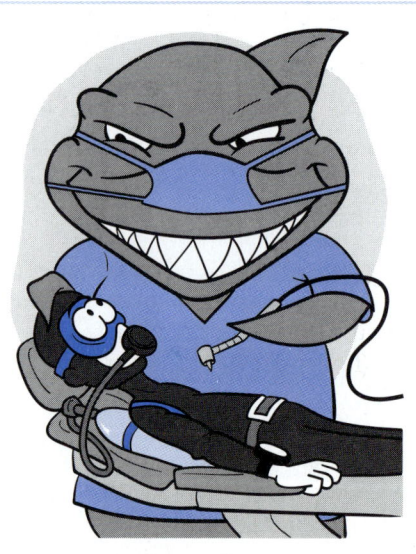

What if . . .

Your diving companion has severe tooth pain?

You're SCUBA diving and suddenly your companion develops severe tooth pain. Is this a coincidence? Is it the consequence of too much candy and not enough flossing? Well, don't be surprised if it's related to the SCUBA diving. One of the most well-known problems related to SCUBA diving is decompression illness (DCI), commonly referred to as "the bends." However, there are several other problems related to SCUBA diving, including air gas embolism (AGE), gas-related breathing problems, and barotrauma.

You may recall Boyle's Law, which tells us that, at a constant temperature, a gas's volume is inversely proportionate to the pressure exerted on that gas. When SCUBA diving, pressure increases with your increase in depth; gases in your body are subject to that pressure. Increasing pressure decreases gas volume. The pressure of 33′ of sea water (fsw), is the equivalent of 2 atmospheres of pressure and 3 atmospheres at 66 fsw. Conversely, during your ascent from the depths, pressure decreases and the volume of gases in your body increases. If the increase in gas volume is too rapid, you can experience pain related to that increase. The pain caused by these pressure and volume changes is called *barotrauma*.

At this point, you're probably asking, "What in the world does that have to do with a toothache?" Occasionally, when a dentist drills and fills a cavity, air gets trapped underneath the material used for the filling. This air is subject to contraction and expansion with pressure changes and a rapid decrease in pressure can create a rapid increase in volume of the gas trapped under the filling causing dental barotrauma, or mechanical pressure within the tooth, which can be painful. In fact, some people have reported needing a root canal after diving.

What To Do

Causes of tooth pain vary, depending on when the person experiences the pain.

Ups...

If the tooth pain has developed during the ascent to the surface from a dive, it may be due to the mouthpiece aggravating the nerve root of an unhealthy tooth or another dental problem unrelated to diving; however, it's most likely due to dental barotrauma. If you're still in the ascent process, slow it down. If your air supply safely allows, dive deeper than the depth when the pain began, then slowly return to the surface. It's generally recommended that your ascent be at a rate of no more than 30' per minute and that you execute a safety stop at 15' to 20'. While the pain is present and when it's safe and convenient to do so, tap the teeth that might be affected and try to identify which tooth is the culprit so, when you get to a dentist, you can tell him exactly which tooth is hurting.

If the pain developed during your ascent, but your companion didn't report it until out of the water and on your way back home, pain relievers, such as acetaminophen, are in order. If the tooth has a filling (dental restoration), then dental barotrauma is most likely. Dental pain with diving has also been reported in recently placed crowns or may be a sign of an affected root that needs a root canal. If the pain persists, a trip to the dentist may be necessary.

 WARNING!!! Make sure the dentist replaces fillings instead of extracting the tooth unnecessarily. Dental barotrauma is caused by air trapped underneath the filling, so the filling should be replaced with careful attention to avoid such air entrapment.

. . . and downs

Tooth pain during the descent portion of a dive may not be coming from an affected tooth. The pain may be referred pain from another location affected by pressure changes, such as the maxillary sinuses. People with chronic or low-grade acute sinusitis can experience pain in the upper dental arch. Looking for other clinical signs of sinusitis can help sort this out. Past history of sinusitis, purulent or bloody nasal discharge, and reproducible pain by exerting pressure over the sinus areas of the face are all clinical clues to the presence of sinusitis.

Prevention and Preparation

As with so many problems from diving, the key to prevention is controlled gradual ascent from the depths. An ascent rate of less than 30′ per minute is generally recommended and a safety stop is wise at a depth of 15′ to 20′. A person should avoid diving if they know they have dental problems. For example, if you have had an intermittently painful tooth, you're recovering from an abscessed tooth or recent root canal, or you have a temporary crown in place while waiting for your permanent crown to be placed, you should avoid a diving expedition or advise your friend to avoid a diving expedition.

To prepare for possible medical problems while diving, check out the Divers Alert Network website at *http://www.diversalertnetwork.org.*

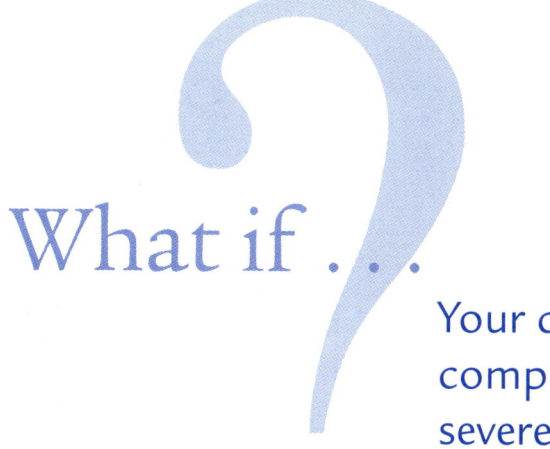

What if . . .

Your diving companion has severe vertigo?

Divers may experience vertigo and nausea, sometimes accompanied by vomiting. If you notice your diving companion is spinning in the water or struggling to orient his body, it's likely that he's suffering from vertigo. When vertigo occurs without ear pain or hearing loss, it's less serious and is most likely due to a disorder related to barotrauma known as *alternobaric vertigo*. Alternobaric vertigo occurs typically during ascent and is attributed to unequal pressures between the right and left middle ears. If the diver is wearing a full wetsuit, the vertigo may be caused by pulling the hood away from the side of his head and allowing cold water to rush into his ear. This temperature-induced vertigo will resolve quickly and isn't of concern.

What To Do

At the first sign of vertigo during diving, a diver should take precautions to prevent progression, prevent further barotrauma to the ear, and prevent consequences of the vertigo. Very gently attempt to equalize ear pressures. Valsalva's maneuver should be performed very gently with low pressure. Even better, have your friend swallow and flex the muscles of the pharynx to open the eustachian tubes gently. A forceful Valsalva's maneuver may cause the rupture of a tympanic membrane or labyrinthine window.

 WARNING!!! If a diver is experiencing alternobaric vertigo, clearly one of his eustachian tubes isn't functioning as well as the other, so further diving puts the diver at increased risk of increased barotrauma injury to the structures of the ear.

Stay with your companion and accompany him to the surface in a controlled, safe ascent. When out of the water, have your companion lie still with his eyes open until the vertigo resolves. Although alternobaric vertigo is self-limiting and usually fairly transient, there can be serious consequences.

 WARNING!!! Divers can become disoriented and also may have severe vomiting. Disorientation and vomiting under water are events associated with an increased risk of drowning.

If the vertigo resolves soon after surfacing, don't let your companion resume diving. His eustachian tube function is clearly not up to par. If the vertigo doesn't resolve within a reasonable period of time or if there is hearing loss associated with the vertigo, he'll need a thorough evaluation by an ENT physician. Very rarely, persistent vertigo may be due to a form of decompression-related illness. (*Please note:* There are other forms of diving-related vertigo associated with diving to extreme depths that require special mixtures of gases such as helium. These extreme diving problems are beyond the scope of this book.)

Prevention and Preparation

Frequently equalize ear pressures during diving by using the methods previously described. Avoid diving if you're suffering from conditions that compromise the function of your eustachian tubes, such as upper respiratory infections and allergic rhinitis. If you have had ear surgery, you shouldn't be diving without the permission of your ENT physician.

Notes

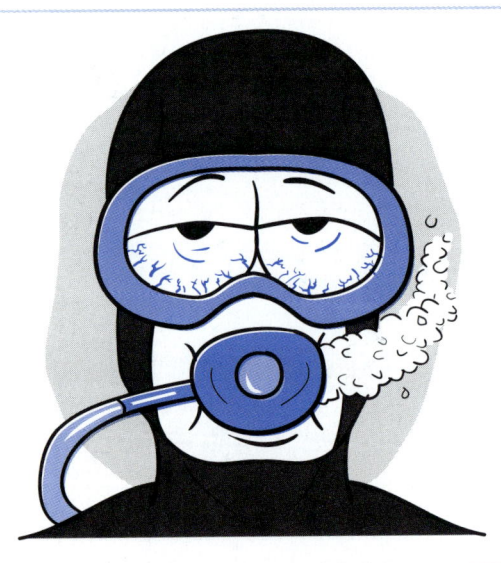

What if . . . Your diving companion has subconjunctival hemorrhages?

It isn't unusual to see someone with subconjunctival hemorrhages after diving, especially a novice diver. This injury is usually the consequence of a phenomenon commonly known as *mask squeeze*. Mask squeeze happens as a diver descends. The increasing pressure creates an effect inside the diving mask that is the equivalent of a partial vacuum. This effect may cause capillary ruptures that result in subconjunctival hemorrhages and petechiae of the peri-orbital skin. It may also cause a red ring on the face in the same shape as the perimeter of the diving mask or even ecchymoses around the eyes.

What To Do

Don't panic! This looks much worse than it is. It isn't a serious injury and will resolve on its own. However, it may take several weeks to resolve completely. Nevertheless, take the time to examine the affected eye or eyes carefully. Subconjunctival hemorrhages will spread across the surface of the sclera, underneath the conjunctival membrane, but won't redden the ciliary border of the iris. If a ciliary flush or inflammation of the border of the iris is present, then something else is going on. Most likely it's an iritis and has nothing to do with subconjunctival hemorrhage but should be examined and treated by an ophthalmologist as soon as possible. Make sure you ask your companion about other symptoms that could be worrisome, such as visual loss, seeing flashing lights, or eye pain.

> WARNING!!! If the hemorrhages or petechiae are accompanied by eye pain, loss of vision, flashing lights, or the appearance of a curtainlike effect in your vision, the victim may be suffering more serious barotrauma to the eye such as a retinal detachment and must be taken to an ophthalmologist for thorough evaluation.

Performing a thorough eye examination and asking these questions will help you pinpoint the diagnosis. What's more, doing so will also make your friend feel more comfortable when you reassure him that, although a subconjunctival hemorrhage may look serious, it isn't.

Prevention and Preparation

The best way to prevent mask squeeze is to periodically puff some air into your mask during your descent into the depths. If you're scuba diving, even as a novice, you're required to take a course and be certified to dive. This prevention method is typically taught in a certification course, but it's easy for a novice to forget when worrying about more complex matters in the process of scuba diving. Being aware of your companion's diving experience level and instructing when necessary on some of the basics can help prevent this *What if* from squeezing the fun out of your dive.

What if . . . Your diving companion becomes ill the day after diving?

Diving-related decompression illness (DCI) may have an onset of symptoms up to 72 hours after a dive episode (and an incident after 96 hours has been reported). Mild DCI may have vague, almost flulike symptoms, that include headache, muscle ache, and fatigue. Symptoms related to other problems not related to DCI are addressed in other *What if* entries on pages 277 and 281.

Signs and symptoms of DCI include myalgia and arthralgia, pruritus and skin blotchiness, muscle weakness or paralysis, numbness or paresthesias, difficulty urinating, tremors, hemoptysis, shortness of breath, and collapse to unconsciousness. DCI is usually categorized as:

- *decompression sickness (DCS),* which is mostly due to dissolved nitrogen gas in tissues reforming gas bubbles and expanding and has signs and symptoms that include paresthesias and myalgia (most common), muscle weakness, and inability to void.
- *air gas embolism (AGE),* which is due to rapid ascent from the depths, causing the formation of nitrogen bubbles in the blood stream that embolize into small arteries, commonly in the central nervous system, and has signs and symptoms that are more severe and neurologic or

pulmonary in nature, including seizure, loss of consciousness, disorientation, stroke, severe chest pain, respiratory arrest, and death.

What To Do

If oxygen is available, administer it to the victim and get the victim to the nearest emergency facility. If no facilities are nearby, contact the Divers Alert Network (DAN). If no telephone is available, keep the victim calm and at rest but transport her to the nearest medical facility.

 WARNING!!! Be alert to illnesses that develop after diving. If the person feels fine the day of and the day after diving but then exercises heavily or takes an airplane flight and subsequently becomes ill, suspect DCI!

On rare occasions, a person who has recently been diving may notice subcutaneous emphysema, particularly in the area above the clavicles or at the base of the neck. This is likely not serious and may be due to an overly aggressive Valsalva's maneuver while trying to clear the eustachian tubes. It may also represent mild pulmonary barotraumas. The person should have a medical evaluation to determine the cause of the subcutaneous emphysema because it may not be diving-related.

Epistaxis, sinus pain, or purulent nasal drainage may be a sign of underlying chronic or acute sinusitis. However, it may be due to diving-related barotrauma, in which air is trapped in the sinuses and causes damage to the mucosal blood vessels. This condition should resolve over time, but be alert to the development of a secondary sinus infection.

Prevention and Preparation

The incidence of DCI can be reduced by using dive tables or computer-based dive tables, available through DAN, the U.S. Navy, SCUBA, and other sources. Diving requires professional training and certification. No one should SCUBA dive without being trained and certified. In using dive tables, experienced divers commonly use a table depth that is greater than the planned diving depth as a conservative measure.

Also note that flying or traveling to high altitudes soon after diving increases the risk of DCI, so don't do it. DAN has a guide for flying after diving. A diver should relax and breathe normally during an ascent, being sure to exhale to avoid trapping air in the lung tissue.

In addition, also consider some general principles to prevent diving-related illnesses:

- Try to keep in good physical condition.
- Avoid heavy exercise before, during, or after diving.
- Avoid dehydration.
- Avoid excessive alcohol intake before and after dives and don't dive with a severe "hangover."
- Keep your ascension rate at 30′ per minute or slower and use a safety stop at about 15′ of depth for about 4 or 5 minutes. Extra caution during ascension (and at all times when diving) is necessary if you're over 40 years of age, obese, or have chronic health problems.

Suffice it to say, SCUBA diving is not a sport for the person with a passing fancy about being underwater. It's a serious sport that requires good technical training; physical training; and attention to detail before, during, and after a dive.

What if . . .

You or a friend falls through the ice?

There are numerous opportunities for this *What if* scenario to happen to anyone. Thousands of people each year are out ice skating, fishing, cross-country skiing, snowmobiling, trying to rescue a dog that has run out onto thin ice and fallen through. Even when it seems logical that the ice should be frozen solid enough to hold your weight or that of your vehicle, it's hard to predict currents or turbulence that cause irregularities in ice formation.

What To Do

Stay calm and don't panic. Concentrate initially on keeping your head above water and breathing. You have fallen into ice water. The initial response is one of gasping and hyperventilation, commonly referred to as *cold shock*. Control your activity. Gasping with your head under water may turn you into a drowning victim. The hyperventilation may cause hypocapnia, hypertension, and tachycardia, which may even lead to myocardial infarction (especially if you have underlying coronary artery disease). This cold immersion response will go away, so concentrate on not drowning and controlling your breathing. If your friend has fallen through the ice, yell these same instructions in simple terms;

say, "Stay calm! Stay still! Control your breathing! We'll get you out!"

Over the following 2 to 15 minutes you'll be subjected to the effects of severe peripheral cooling, which leads to slowing and weakening neuromuscular activity. Your hands and fingers will stiffen up, your movements will become less coordinated. This span of time is actually a reasonable amount to save yourself or get help. Before this effect severely incapacitates you, position yourself so that you're facing the direction you came from when you fell in. (Presumably, the ice you were on just before you fell in was strong enough to support your weight.) Place your arms onto the ice surface and kick your feet in order to get your body as horizontal as possible, making it easier for you to kick and pull yourself onto the ice surface and out of the ice water. Once onto the ice, roll yourself away from the ice hole. While executing these maneuvers, yell repeatedly for help. There may be someone nearby who can help rescue you. Stay horizontal and crawl your way to more solid ice or dry ground.

If you're initially unsuccessful with these maneuvers, repeat them and don't forget to keep yelling for help. Over the next 15 to 60 minutes, you'll experience core temperature cooling that will eventually lead to unconsciousness.

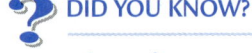

DID YOU KNOW?

More time than you think

It's commonly thought that you'll die within a few minutes if you fall through the ice. In fact, as long as you don't panic and succumb from gasping water into your lungs or hyperventilating yourself into a myocardial infarction, you have more time than you think. You actually have at least 10 minutes before you lose your ability to perform meaningful physical maneuvers, such as pulling yourself from the ice hole. You then have about an hour before serious hypothermia sets in. So, if you have at least positioned yourself with your arms on the surface of the ice, you have time for someone to come to your rescue.

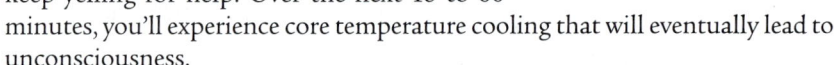

WARNING!!! If your friend has fallen in, don't become the next victim! You can't help your friend if you fall through the ice, too. Shout to your friend the instructions previously described. Don't venture to the edge of the ice hole. Use a device such as a rope or long tree branch or even an article of clothing (such as a jacket) as a rescue tool that your friend can grab onto and you can use to help pull him out of the water. Only venture as far onto the ice as is necessary to get the rescue tool to your friend. If you have a rope, tie a loop in the end so that it's easier for your friend to grab onto or loop around his arm.

THE FINAL MOVE THAT MAY SAVE YOUR LIFE

If the kicking and pulling maneuver has failed to get you out of the ice hole, position your arms and body as far onto the ice surface as you can. Do this when you feel you have no additional strength or capacity to be repeating the maneuver. Stay in that position as long as you can maintain consciousness. With a little bit of luck, the wet sleeves of your clothing will freeze and adhere to the surface of the ice, keeping your head above water if you lose consciousness. This maneuver gives you the longest period of time for potential rescue by someone else who happens by or has heard your cries for help.

Escape from the Ice

When you've successfully escaped from the water and onto dry ground, the next challenge is to begin warming yourself and drying out. If you're a long way from help and are stranded, you'll need to build a fire as soon as possible. With the fire built, stay close to stay warm, and try removing some of your wet clothing in order to dry it out near the fire. Perhaps start with your jacket or even your shirt followed by your jacket. Once dry, put the article of clothing on and remove other wet clothing to dry. Obviously, if it's your friend who has fallen through the ice, clothe him in some of your dry clothing while his clothing is drying out by the fire.

Prevention and Preparation

If you're planning an ice expedition, such as snowmobiling or cross-country skiing, know the ice conditions. Get accurate information from local authorities. Take rescue equipment with you in a backpack attached to you. The pack should also include waterproof fire starting materials. Also, use the buddy system: ski, skate, or fish with a buddy. Snowmobile with someone else on their snowmobile. Of course, before you venture out onto the ice, take a moment to think about what you'll do if this *What if* happens to you or a friend.

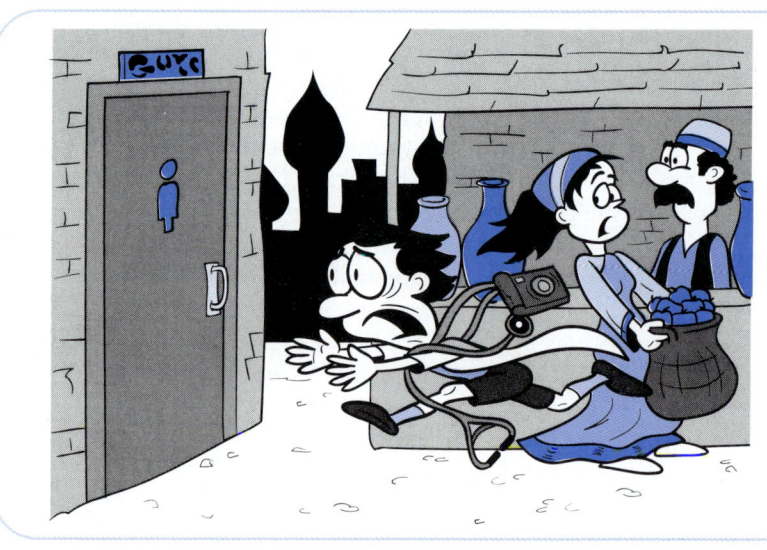

What if . . .

You or your friend develops diarrhea in a foreign country?

Diarrhea: the bane of all travelers. Who wants to have a trip spoiled by sitting on the toilet instead of enjoying the culinary delights of a new place? Fortunately, diarrhea is preventable and treatable.

Traveler's diarrhea is characterized by an increase in the frequency of unformed bowel movements (usually four to five) associated with abdominal cramping, vomiting, bloating, and malaise. More severe symptoms include fever and bloody diarrhea. The diarrhea may occur during travel or soon after returning home and is usually self-limited. Although rarely persistent, the illness can last 3 to 4 days and more than one episode may occur during the same trip.

The most important determinant of risk is the destination of the traveler. Higher-risk destinations where the attack risk reaches almost 50% are South America, Africa, the Middle East, Asia, southern Europe, and a few Caribbean islands. The main culprit in traveler's diarrhea is the ingestion of stool contaminated food or water, such as undercooked meat or seafood, raw fruits and vegetables, tap water, and unpasteurized dairy products. These foods transmit infectious bacterial, viral, and parasitic organisms that cause symptoms by invading the mucosal lining of the intestine or producing toxins. Common transmitted agents are *Escherichia coli, Shigella, Giardia, Cryptosporidium,* hepatitis A, *Campylobacter,* and Norwalk virus.

What To Do

Because most traveler's diarrhea is self-limited, the most important treatment is drinking fluids that replace the salts lost through the diarrhea to prevent dehydration. The World Health Organization makes an oral rehydration salt solution packet that can be purchased at most stores and pharmacies and prepared by adding one packet to boiled or treated water. This salt solution contains sodium chloride, potassium chloride, glucose, and trisodium citrate, and should be consumed in small amounts frequently for the duration of symptoms. Other adequate replacement fluids include carbonated beverages, such as sports drinks and ginger ale, and chicken broth.

 WARNING!!! Drinking only pure water doesn't replace any of the salts lost through the diarrhea and may cause weakness, mental status changes, and even seizures if consumed excessively.

Several over-the-counter agents have been used to limit the frequency and duration of symptoms. Bismuth subsalicylate (Pepto-Bismol) may shorten the duration of the illness and decrease the frequency of the diarrhea. Antimotility agents, loperamide (Imodium) and diphenoxylate (Lomotil), slow stool transit through the intestine.

 WARNING!!! Patients with kidney problems should limit their use of Pepto-Bismol because large amounts of bismuth may concentrate in the kidneys, causing renal failure. Loperamide and diphenoxylate are

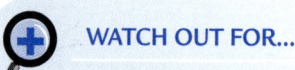 **WATCH OUT FOR...**

Three common travel diseases

There are some common diarrhea-related diseases that are typically acquired during travel. Three of these diseases are described.

Giardiasis

Giardiasis is commonly acquired while trekking or backpacking in rural areas. Because its incubation period is 1 to 3 weeks, symptoms generally appear after returning from travel and, thus, the disease isn't always thought of as travel-related. The infection typically persists until diagnosed and treated. Enzyme Immunoassay for Giardia Specific Antigen is the best diagnostic test, as stool is intermittently positive for ova or parasites. Standard treatment in the U.S. has been metronidazole, but more recently tinidazole and nitazoxanide have become available.

Cryptosporidiosis

Cryptosporidiosis is increasingly prevalent in the U.S. and

foreign countries and is usually picked up in hotel swimming pools (because it's resistant to chlorine treatment). Symptoms appear from 2 to 10 days after ingestion and last up to 2 weeks; however, a carrier state can persist for months. Treatment has typically been azithromycin; however, nitazoxanide is now available in the U.S. and is considered 90 percent effective.

Fish-borne illnesses

Look out for some fish-borne illnesses that include diarrhea among their symptom complex. For example, ciguatoxin may be found in barracuda and tropical reef fish. In addition to the diarrheal illness, neurologic symptoms such as temperature reversal, weakness, and pain sensitivity are also associated with this type of illness. In addition, scombroid poisoning is caused by tuna, mackerel, bonito, and mahi-mahi. High histamine levels in these fish cause flushing, nausea, vomiting, diarrhea, and urticaria.

contraindicated in patients with high fever or bloody stools because they may worsen problems associated with enterotoxin-producing bacterial infections, especially without accompanying antimicrobial therapy.

Antimicrobial agents have also been used to treat and prevent traveler's diarrhea. Currently, the Centers for Disease Control and Prevention recommends against using antibiotic prophylaxis to prevent diarrhea. However, antibiotics may be useful for diarrhea that persists more than 3 to 4 days or is associated with bloody stools, high fever, persistent vomiting, and shaking chills. Antimicrobial therapy may shorten the duration of symptoms, particularly if the offending agent is sensitive to the drug. The most effective and commonly used antibiotic is ciprofloxacin (500 mg) taken twice daily for 3 days. Antibiotics shouldn't be used without a consultation with a physician.

Prevention and Preparation

To avoid travelers diarrhea, limit your exposure to contaminated food and water. Here are some tips on how to do just that.

Avoid Dangers

Here are some dangers to avoid that might expose your body to contamination:

- Raw or undercooked meats and seafood
- Raw fruits and vegetables unless the skin can be peeled
- Beverages purchased from street vendors or those with ice made from tap water
- Unpasteurized milk and dairy products

Practice Safety

Practice safe eating habits when in a foreign country, including:

- Eating properly handled, well-cooked food or packaged foods
- Eating raw fruit or vegetables that you can peel yourself
- Boiling your water for a minute or so and drinking carbonated, bottled beverages; boiled water; or teas
- Using carbonated bottled water for drinking and brushing teeth

Cyber Travel First

Prepare for the inevitable challenges of traveling in a strange land. Some useful websites to peruse when planning your trip abroad include:

- *http://www.cdc.gov/travel/*—The CDC provides up-to-date health warnings and general practical information for travelers by destination.
- *http://www.who.int/en*—The World Health Organization provides updated health hazards by country.
- *http://travel.state.gov/*—This site is useful for general travel information, such as safety warnings and visa requirements.

Index

A

B

C

D

E

F

G

H

Q

R

S

Tinnitus, and syncope, 7
Tiredness, 67–69
Tooth pain, in divers, 277–279
Tourniquet, for bleeding patient, 216
    for patient with catheter broken in vein, 78
    for snakebite victim, 233
Transference, 151
Trauma. *See particular injury types (e.g.,* Bites;
    Fractures*) and site-specific entries.*
Traveler's diarrhea, 295–298
Treatment, refusal of, 187–189
    by child's parents, 199
Tree-pit snow shelter, 245
Tuning fork test, for loss of sensation, 165
Tympanic membrane injury, examination for,
    83–84
Tyrannical behavior, 57–60

U

Ultrasonography, in imaging of obese patient,
    96
Umbilical cord, unraveling of, in delivery, 104,
    105
Underwater divers. *See* SCUBA divers.
Upper arm splint, 259
Upper respiratory tract manifestations, of al-
    lergic reactions, 135
Uterine contractions, and delivery, 103

V

Vaccine, hepatitis, for health-care workers, 80
Vagal activity, and syncope, 7
Vehicular injuries, management of, 115–118
Vengeful behavior, 59
Venomous snakes, 191, 232
    bites by, 191, 192, 231–233
Venous catheter placement, complications of,
    77–78
Venous cutdown, imaging as aid to, in obese
    patient, 96
Ventilation, for newborn, 110
Ventricular fibrillation, 129
    management of, 100, 129–132
Vertigo, in divers, 281–282

Viagra (sildenafil), for altitude sickness, 226
Vibratory sensation test, 165
Violence, gun-related, 93–94
    patient engaging in or threatening, 17–19,
    177–178
Viral hepatitis, transmission of, via needle-
    stick, 79, 80
Visually impaired patient, communication
    with, 35–37

W

Walking, assisting blind patient with, 36
Warmer, for injected solutions, 174
Warming, of frostbite victim, 250
    of newborn, 105
    of victim of ice-water immersion, 293
Water, as target for lightning, 255–256
    contaminated, 241, 296–297
    dangers of diving in. *See specifics under*
      SCUBA divers.
    disinfection of, 240
    fresh, sources of, 240
      pathogens in, 241
    immersion in, fall through ice and, 291–293
    infectious organisms in, 241, 296–297
    irrigation of ear with, 84
    jellyfish hazards in, 273–274
    outdoor sources of, 240–241
    purification of, 240
Weapon(s), dealing with patient possessing,
    18, 91–92
    emergencies involving, 93–94
Wilderness injuries, 215–218
Work, faking of illness for excuse from, 163
    request for excuse from, 185
Written communication, with deaf patient, 32

X

X-ray studies, in imaging of obese patient, 96

Z

Zero tolerance, for violence, 19
Zidovudine, in postexposure prophylaxis for
    HIV infection, 80